ALSO BY JOE BOVINO

For even faster and more remarkable results, order Joe Bovino's complete Sugar Belly Secret weight-loss system.

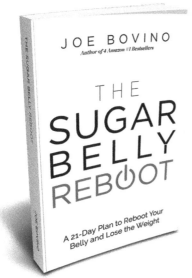

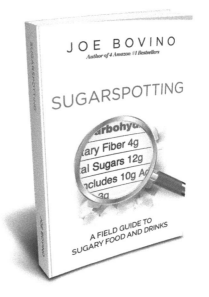

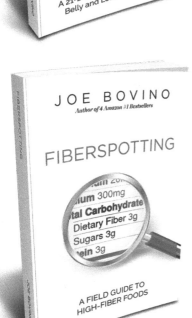

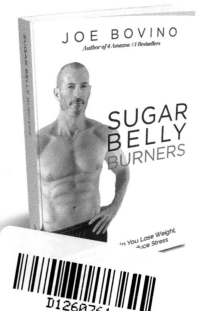

Available only at

www.TheSugarBellySecret.com

THE
SUGAR
BELLY
SECRET

Subtract the Sugar, Lose the Weight, and Transform Your Life

JOE BOVINO

Printed in the United States of America

First Printing, 2018

Published by Book Counselor, LLC

Bookcounselor.com

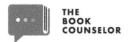

THE
BOOK
COUNSELOR

Table of Contents

Introduction

How the mighty had fallen.

In 2004, at the age of 41, I became known as Joe Bovino from P90X (aka "P90X Joe," "Tony's twin," or "Triceps boy"), the most popular extreme home workout program in the world.

Celebrities and politicians were trying P90X and heard my full name because Tony Horton, the fitness trainer behind the program and an old buddy of mine, says it about 10 times during the Shoulders & Arms workout, where I appear as a cast member.

People started recognizing me everywhere—and not just in the United States. They treated me like royalty, even in places like Moscow, Russia. (I explained that I wasn't Tony Horton, but they didn't care. I appeared in P90X. That was good enough for them.)

The company that produced P90X hired me to appear in one of the videos because I participated in a test group for the product and crushed it. P90X legitimately transformed my body, aesthetically at least, and I loved sporting a 6-pack for the first time.

But the story doesn't end there because… my results didn't last for long.

I couldn't sustain it.

Few people who try P90X, or any other exercise program for that matter, can. It's just too hard, time-consuming, monotonous, or inconvenient; something else almost always happens that results in a setback.

The same goes for most new diets, gym memberships, and even weight-loss surgeries.

Bad habits return, and so does the weight.

We've all watched Oprah, Kirstie Alley, and other celebrities yo-yo from fat to not-so-fat and back again despite access to expensive personal trainers and nutritionists. It's embarrassing, but it sheds light on a dirty little secret about most of these diets and fitness programs: Most people see changes at the start as their bodies adapt to a positive intervention but inevitably drift back to where they started, only now they're more cynical, frustrated, and disappointed.

In my case, I regained all of my pre-P90X weight, watched my waistline expand and abs disappear, lost muscle, and experienced a rapid decline in overall health and fitness.

I tried to recover with more 90-day rounds of P90X and even started an online workout support group to stay focused, but the pendulum swung back to mediocrity every time.

I went from P90X Joe to Average Joe.

My bad habits and age weren't just catching up to me. They were winning.

Then, in 2012 at the age of 49, the wheels really fell off.

I was holding my own in a yoga class full of fit women, including my beautiful date for the day whom I thought might be a keeper if she'd stop calling me and everyone else "babe." (That was annoying, but I digress....)

Then, as I completed the last sit-up and stood for a few parting words, chants, or heavy breathing, the world started spinning before my eyes like a movie in fast forward.

I didn't know what the f-ck was happening. I couldn't even remember which direction I was facing. The room was as hot as a sauna, but I suddenly felt cold and extremely nauseous.

Only one thing made sense—sit down before I fall on my face.

I'd also scarfed down four pieces of Kentucky Fried Chicken before class and desperately didn't want to see it again. Please, God, no. Not now.

I closed my eyes to make the spinning stop, but it didn't work, at least not right away. The movie played on in my head like a spinning nightmare.

I just sat there, sweating profusely and white as a ghost, trying to ride it out.

By the time I could stand up with a little help from my friends, I was a wreck. I looked and moved like an old man at death's door.

It was humiliating, embarrassing and, frankly, scary.

The yoga teacher asked if she should call an ambulance. I said "No thank you. I'll be fine," but I wasn't fine. Eventually, my date escorted me back to my apartment in the same complex … one baby step at a time.

I sat on the sofa and tried to convince her (and myself) that I wasn't a complete p-ssy. Then, still worried that I might hurl and ruin everything, I shuffled to the kitchen, grabbed the Tums, took a few, and sat down again.

Bad idea. Almost instantaneously, my fear of losing control again became a reality. I barely made it to the toilet before vomiting furiously into it, while my date sat horrified in the other room, occasionally asking "Are you OK, babe?"

When I finally emerged from the bathroom, I was a shell of the man I was only a few hours earlier, and I reluctantly agreed that she should call 911.

The paramedics arrived in minutes, wheeled me out on a stretcher, and took me to the emergency room of a local hospital, where nurses hooked me up to machines and ran a few tests.

While I laid there recovering, two people died in beds across the room. I'm not kidding. They covered 'em up and wheeled 'em away, just like on TV.

Finally, a doctor showed up to relay the results of my tests, but when I asked him about the diagnosis, all he could say was, "You had vertigo."

That's it? Of course I had vertigo, you dope! I knew that already.

What I needed to know was *why* I had vertigo and *how* to prevent it from happening again, but he didn't have a clue, and neither did I when they sent me home.

I was supposed to spend the rest of my life worrying about my next attack and avoiding activities that could trigger one.

The prospect of living like that upset me for many reasons, including the massive blow to my confidence, appearance, and health, not to mention the likely impact on my bachelor life.

High-quality single women weren't looking for a guy on his last legs, if you will, and I wasn't surprised when my date for yoga class stopped returning my calls. I never saw her again.

She found another babe, I guess.

How could this be happening to *me*?

Was I supposed to accept a life of middle-age mediocrity without a fight?

No f-cking way.

If the doctors weren't going to give me any useful guidance or otherwise help me get my sh-t together, I'd take matters into my own hands.

The Search for Answers

The first thing I did was take a hard look at my diet.

I knew from years of experience in health and fitness, including a couple spent training alongside famous bodybuilders, athletes, and actors at

Gold's Gym in Venice, CA, that at least 80% of success in losing weight and getting fit depends on one's diet, not exercise.

Plus, whenever I attempted another round of P90X or any other strenuous exercise program, my vertigo returned, albeit not as badly, and ended the workout fast. It occasionally tormented me when I wasn't exercising, too. I'd be walking down the street, lose my balance for no apparent reason, and wonder what the f-ck was happening to me.

The answers I needed didn't come right away by any means.

I experimented with all kinds of diets–low-carb, high-carb, low-fat, juicing, vegan, gluten-free, Mediterranean, and weight-loss systems comprised of some combination thereof. I read books and watched videos by leading experts in the field too, including Dr. Richard Jacoby, Dr. Robert Lustig, Dave Zinczenko, Gary Taubes and others about the dangers of sugar.

It took years and a lot of patience, but as I struggled to discern which diet (and complementary exercise training regimen) was superior, I discovered something surprising: Despite drawbacks of various kinds with the most popular low-carb diets, including major sustainability problems, most of them worked in the short-term if they were executed properly... but so did many of the high-carb diets.

This baffling revelation complicated and significantly delayed my decision about the best way forward, but it also raised an important question...

How can low-carb *and* high-carb diets work?

How is that even possible, especially when they tend to point the finger at each other?

What do they have in common?

Is there a way to reconcile the differences, take the best, and forget the rest?

Yes, there is.

When you cut through all the noise and hyperbole, all successful diets do three things:

1. Subtract sugar,
2. Add fiber, and
3. Subtract alcohol.

That's the Sugar Belly Secret, folks.

If you're slightly more daring, you can double down by adding exercise (and more sleep) for even more remarkable results. That's what I do, and I hope you'll join me for some simple, belly-busting workouts someday, but it's not necessary. Exercise is optional.

The Sugar Belly Secret isn't a "diet" in the traditional sense, but that's the beauty of it. Diets are too complicated. All you have to do is add and subtract: Subtract the excess sugar and alcohol that come in processed, fake or toxic products and add the fiber that comes in real, healthy ones.

It's a proven, natural way to lose your sugar belly *for good*, maintain and build fat-burning muscle, and improve your overall health and fitness without counting calories, carbs or healthy fats, watching portion sizes, or even exercising.

Pretty simple, right?

Not so fast.

The Food and Beverage industries, in conjunction with the sugar lobby, grocery and restaurant industries, have effectively processed, reformulated, adulterated, tainted (and, according to some experts, poisoned) our food supply so thoroughly that it's incredibly hard to avoid consuming fiberless food with added sugar and getting fat.

They've also stifled efforts by the FDA and other organizations to increase transparency about the amount of added sugar in our food and beverages by delaying implementation of a new nutrition label that would have helped us to make more informed decisions as consumers by requiring companies to reveal the total "added sugars" in their products.

I hate to say it, but they want you in the dark. It will cost a lot of money to make many of their products healthier once consumers wise up and explore alternatives, and most companies aren't interested in relabeling their products, either.

Meanwhile, the U.S. government has been reluctant to rock the boat by at least requiring more transparency for fear of losing political contributions and tax dollars, and some agencies have acted like willing accomplices, wittingly or unwittingly.

The party line goes like this: If you develop a sugar belly, get sick, spend years in ill health, or die young because you consume too many processed foods and drinks, it's your fault and problem, not theirs. Most of these companies, organizations and agencies aren't even willing to help you make more fully informed decisions.

It's up to you to educate yourself, understand what's going on behind the scenes, and take action.

The costs of not doing so are serious—even deadly—and growing rapidly, along with your waistline.

A new, comprehensive study by the Institute of Health Metrics and Evaluation at the University of Washington concluded that a bad diet now causes one in five deaths, with obesity the fastest growing global risk. Diet is also the second highest risk factor for early death, after smoking.

Similarly, according to a new report by the Centers for Disease Control and Prevention, forty percent (40%) of all cancer diagnoses in the United

States are now linked to excess weight, including more than half (55%) of all cancers diagnosed in women.

I wrote this book to help you understand the sugar belly debacle, lose weight, and stay healthy by: (a) spotting and subtracting sugar in all kinds of food and beverages, much of which has been deliberately hidden from you; (b) spotting and adding fiber, much of which has been removed from food against your interests; and (c) spotting and subtracting alcoholic beverages that are keeping you fat, sick, and troubled.

It worked for me once I discovered the Sugar Belly Secret, and it still does.

Today, at the age of 55, I'm arguably stronger and healthier than I was after my first round of P90X fourteen years ago, and I've been able to sustain my results easily over time.

I'm at the top of my game as I write this, living and working in Medellin, Colombia, surrounded by some of the most fun-loving people you'll ever meet and, oh yeah, some of the most beautiful women in the world.

I'm helping others to lose weight, stay healthy, and get fit, too—in-person, in writing, on video, and online—and I hope this book will spread the word to an even larger audience, starting with you.

And yes, thank God, my vertigo is history. I never found out exactly what caused it or why it disappeared, but I know that taking action to lose my sugar belly and get healthy again made all the difference.

Who knows where I'd be otherwise?

Certainly not in yoga class.

I'm not a physician or a scientist, but I've been extraordinarily active in health and fitness my entire life, learned a great deal as a P90X success story and cast member, and know what it's like to fall apart and bounce back. I came to my conclusions in this book honestly and sincerely through extensive and highly personal research.

I wanted my life back. I wanted to flatten my sugar belly. I wanted to look and feel great for the rest of my life, not some yo-yo BS. And that's what happened.

You can do it too, amigo, no matter how fat, old, sickly or cynical you are right now.

You can beat sugar belly and become the hero of your story.

Or you can ignore or dismiss the wisdom in this book, let the food and beverage industries, sugar lobby, and corrupt politicians continue to deceive and manipulate you, and spend your life flirting with obesity, ill health, and premature death.

(Hell, if you're gonna do that, you might as well start smoking too.)

If you're waiting to be bailed out by a wise politician or bureaucrat, magic weight-loss pill, trendy diet or exercise program, or enlightened food and beverage industry practices, good luck with that.

They won't save you, but it doesn't matter.

You've got this, and I'd be honored to guide you along the way.

All you need is the Sugar Belly Secret and the unvarnished truth about why it works better than anything else, starting with the straight scoop on sugar.

CHAPTER ONE

The Scoop on Sugar

I thought I knew all that I needed to know about sugar.

Boy, was I wrong.

It's not enough to avoid soda, cookies and candy. Not anymore.

Even cutting back on carbs that most people know convert to sugar in your body isn't good enough.

The problem is much bigger than that, and the truth scared me straight.

I hope it does the same for you.

The average American consumes about 160 pounds of sugar each year, or more than 7 ounces per day, including 63 pounds of high-fructose corn syrup ("HFCS"), the most problematic type of added sugar known to cause visceral (intra-organ) fat that wasn't even on the market until 1975.

And that's before taking alcohol consumption into account.

To visualize this more clearly, imagine consuming 27 to 30 teaspoons of sugar *every single day*.

Would you knowingly consume that much sugar if you knew that, while it was expanding your waistline and doubling your chin, it was harming, potentially poisoning, and arguably killing you… slowly but surely?

I don't think you would, not after you get the scoop on added sugar.

You need the ugly truth … so I won't sugar-coat it.

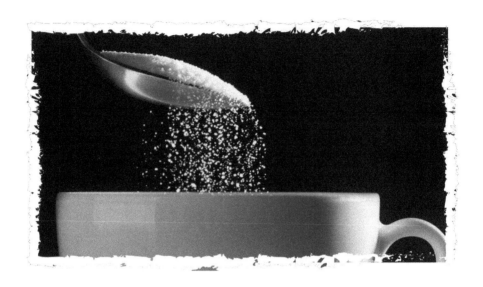

The "Added Sugar" Belly

By now you've no doubt heard the story of America's obesity epidemic, but you may be confused about the villain.

It's not fats. We've reduced our consumption of fats tremendously since 1930, but you wouldn't know that from watching the news.

It's not salt or gluten unless you've got a specific problem in that regard, despite bestselling books claiming otherwise.

It's not carbs generally because many carbs do not make you fat or sick— quite the contrary, as some healthy, high-carb diets have demonstrated.

And it's not you... even if you've made some poor decisions about diet and exercise over the years. Who hasn't? I'm not encouraging a victimization mindset because simply blaming others is an excuse for inaction and resignation in the face of failure, and each of us bears ultimate responsibility for our actions. But we've been spoon-fed fake food and fake news about it for decades, and it's tough to make informed decisions as a consumer under those circumstances.

So, who's the real villain in this story?

You guessed it—processed or added sugar.

When you consume carbs with excessive amounts of added sugar, especially sucrose, fructose, and HFCS in soft drinks, fruit drinks, snacks, and other foods loaded with it, you don't just develop a sugar belly.

You throw your metabolism into a tailspin that leads to a cluster of increasingly common conditions called metabolic syndrome, including obesity, type 2 diabetes, lipid problems, hypertension, and cardiovascular disease, which are causing widespread misery and premature death.

Some experts claim that chronic exposure to added sugar also causes cancer, Alzheimer's, IBS, and other horrible things, and I don't doubt it.

Check out this graph on U.S. sugar consumption from 1822 to 2005:

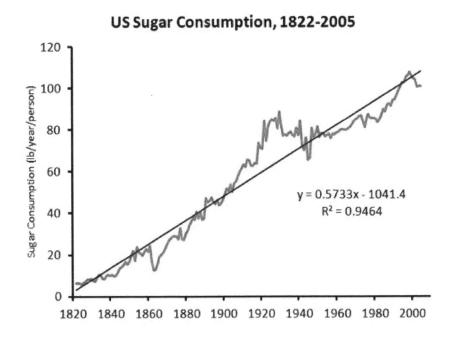

US Sugar Consumption, 1822-2005

$y = 0.5733x - 1041.4$
$R^2 = 0.9464$

Sugar consumption tops out at 120 pounds per person because that was high enough to convey all of the data back in 2005, but we're up to about 160 pounds per person per year in 2017, according to some estimates. So, imagine what the graph looks like today. There have been occasional dips in the trajectory over the last few years, but the upward trend continues largely unabated.

Now, check out this graph on adult obesity rates from 1990 to 2016 in the United States, with one line for each of the 50 states:

Adult obesity rates, 1990 to 2016

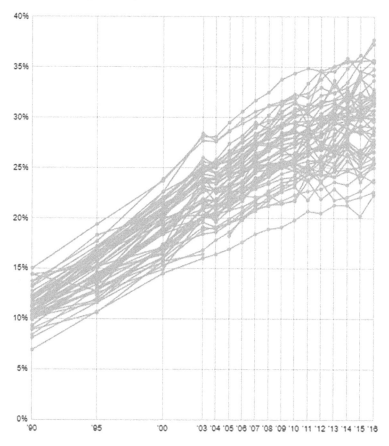

Notice anything about the trajectories of sugar consumption and obesity?

The rate and prevalence of obesity in the United States has skyrocketed along with the amount of sugar consumption, and it's no coincidence.

When these state-by-state results were updated on August 31, 2017, adult obesity rates exceeded 35% in five states (with West Virginia leading the fat pack at 37.7%), 30% in 25 states, and 25% in 46 states (with Colorado bringing up the rear, if you will, at 22.3%).

What does that mean, pound-for-pound?

We weigh about 25% more than we did just 25 years ago, and evidence of our collective chubbiness isn't hard to find or see.

In 1980, only about 15% of American adults were overweight or obese. Now the percentage exceeds 55%; in other words, normal-weight people aren't the norm anymore, and the percentage of overweight and obese adults in the United States is expected to rise to 65% by 2030.

Indeed, most Americans already sport a sugar belly, but don't think you're off the hook if you don't. Studies show that up to 40% of normal-weight adults suffer from a sign of chronic metabolic disease called "insulin resistance." What's that? It's a time bomb waiting to explode on a whole lot of unsuspecting people who incorrectly assume that they're healthy simply because they're not as fat as their neighbor.

Obesity isn't just an American or Western problem anymore, either.

It's a global pandemic.

I feel a sense of pride when American companies succeed internationally and still remember how thrilled I was to see signs and billboards for Coca-Cola, McDonalds, KFC, and other U.S. companies displayed in big cities throughout the former Soviet Union, but as we've tainted our food supply by adding massive amounts of sugar (and removing fiber), we've passed our obesity problem on to the rest of the world, too.

A new study by the prestigious *New England Journal of Medicine* shows that 2.2 billion people (one third of the world's population, with the United States leading the way) are currently overweight or obese.

How did so many people in other countries, who were naturally thin or normal weight for centuries, suddenly join the sugar-belly club?

They consumed a lot more processed food and beverages from the West that are undeniably tasty and relatively inexpensive but tend to be high in sugar and low in fiber.

Fruct' Up

Is all sugar equally bad for you?

No, not really, and it's important to know the difference.

Carbs contain three types of sugar:

1. Glucose
2. Sucrose (table sugar), and
3. Fructose (often in the liquid form of HFCS).

Sucrose is 50% glucose and 50% fructose. HFCS, on the other hand, is up to 55% fructose, tastes sweeter and costs less than sucrose, and comes in a liquid form.

Every cell in your body can metabolize glucose (sometimes affectionately referred to as "the energy of life"), thereby increasing the ability and likelihood of burning it off. But only your liver, which filters toxins (including alcohol), can metabolize fructose, and chronic fructose exposure leads to metabolic syndrome and other serious health problems.

Fructose is a carb, but your body metabolizes it like a fat. That is, your liver responds to fructose by flooding your body with triglycerides (fatty deposits in your blood), which tell your body to store more belly fat, and that's what happens.

In other words, when you consume fructose, you're effectively consuming fat. It's the absolute worst type of sugar for your waistline.

In one research study, subjects consumed beverages sweetened with either glucose or fructose for eight weeks. They gained roughly the same amount of weight by the end of the study, but *anyone who drank fructose gained the weight primarily as sugar-belly fat* because of the way the liver processes it.

Sucrose and HFCS are equally harmful because each delivers fructose to your liver and expands your sugar belly, but HFCS poses more of a problem because its liquid form, extra sweetness, and lower price create an economic incentive for companies to add it surreptitiously to soft drinks, bread, baked goods, snacks, sauce, and, well… you name it.

Before food processing, we consumed fructose by eating fruits and vegetables, but it didn't amount to much, and those foods are packed with fiber and micronutrients that make the trade-off worthwhile… then and now.

But these days, fructose constitutes an absurdly high percentage of the calories that we consume in food and beverages as adults, adolescents, and children. It's off the charts.

Something's gotta give.

Fake News

There's a lot of fake news and quackery about nutrition, but the worst kind relates to low-fat diets (which take your eye off fructose and other added sugars), the expression "a calorie is a calorie," and marketing campaigns designed to make obesity desirable.

'ets Don't Work

For at least 35 years, the U.S. government and many so-called experts on nutrition have been recommending low-fat diets because they purportedly reduce "bad" cholesterol by combating obesity and heart disease.

Unfortunately, they based their conclusions on flawed studies, including an influential 500-page "Seven Countries" one by Ancel Keys in 1980.

Mr. Keys believed that dietary fat was the sole cause of heart disease because of its cholesterol content and tried to prove it. However as Dr. Robert Lustig and other experts on the dangers of sugar have noted, Keys failed to realize that he was actually studying the effects of high-fructose diets, not high-fat diets, because fructose is metabolized like a fat. He also failed to distinguish between two types of low-density lipoproteins ("LDL"). Large buoyant LDL doesn't hurt you; small, dense LDL does.

We know that now, but the food industry responded to the U.S. government's low-fat guidelines back then by introducing all sorts of low-fat foods. And, since low-fat food tastes like Styrofoam, guess what they did? They added sugar to make it palatable, and our rate of sugar consumption and obesity went through the roof.

Since then, so-called low-fat diets have failed miserably. They've created more obesity, illness, and death by opening the door to adulteration of our food supply with processed sugar, and they're not done as long as people continue to peddle and believe fake news about them.

In short, if you like your sugar belly or want a bigger one, go with a low-fat diet. Otherwise, toss them into the trash heap of history, where they belong.

Some Calories Are Better Than Others

If "a calorie is calorie," as some say, then it's up to you to either burn the calories you consume as food or drink, or you will store them as fat.

According to this mantra, if you eat too much or don't exercise enough to burn it off, you're going to get fat.

I'm sure you've heard this well-known concept repeated by food and beverage companies (which don't want to make their products healthier), insurance companies (which need an excuse to deny coverage), doctors (who are often poorly trained in nutrition), gyms (which count on people not showing up), weight loss clinics (which want you as a client), and other companies selling exercise programs and supplements.

Many of these calorie counters recognize that, if you're not satisfied with your results from whatever they're offering, they can always point the finger at you by claiming that you consumed too many calories, didn't exercise enough to burn them off, or both. But it's not that simple because the *quality* of your calories matters as much or more than the quantity.

Calories from healthy complex carbs, proteins, and fats lead to good health, long lives, and flat bellies. Calories from added sugars, fiberless foods, and most alcohol lead to obesity, metabolic disease, and worse.

The distinction couldn't be starker, but we're consuming too many calories from the wrong sources anyway, in part due to caloric relativism.

That needs to change, and there's no time to waste. Forget about counting calories. Make your calories count with the Sugar Belly Secret.

Sorry, but Obesity Isn't Attractive or Desirable

Obesity isn't just unsightly and unappealing to the opposite sex.

It's unhealthy and potentially deadly.

Want to know whether someone is likely to die young?

Look at their waistline.

(Then look at how they walk. If they walk slowly, they typically don't have that many years left. So, put down the pie and pick up the pace!)

Despite these facts, the media and fashion industry frequently try to redefine what it means to be normal, real, cool, beautiful, healthy, or even "evolved" by glorifying overweight women and, to a lesser extent, men.

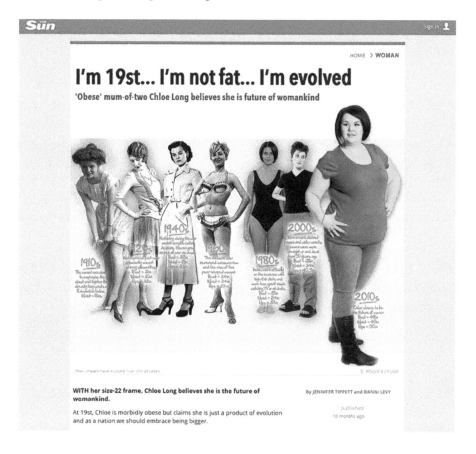

The alternative—noticing the obvious or simply stating the facts—amounts to "fat shaming."

With all due respect, I don't have patience for this kind of political correctness, and neither should you. It's a lie, and it hurts people who believe it by encouraging them to remain fat, unattractive and, more importantly, unhealthy.

All I care about is helping you look better, feel better, and live longer with a sugar-belly breakthrough, and propaganda like this slows us down.

We don't have time for word games and image signaling. We have work to do.

Good News

Are you stuck with your sugar belly, no matter what you do?

No way, even if it feels that way right now.

It's never too late to lose your sugar belly, and it's easier than you think.

This book will show you how by exposing the real problem and setting forth a simple plan to resolve it, starting with an overview of the Game of Hormones going on inside all of us.

If you play the Game smart by subtracting the troublemakers (sugar and alcohol) and adding an underrated peacemaker (fiber), your body will take care of the rest, and your sugar belly will be a thing of the past.

You may lose a few plus-sized modeling gigs, but it's for the best.

CHAPTER 2

Game of Hormones

I went from P9oX Joe to Average Joe by losing a Game of Hormones ("Game") that I didn't even realize I was playing.

But it ain't over 'til the fat lady sings.

Once I figured out how to play the Game, I lost my sugar belly for good.

So can you, but it's hard to win a game that you don't understand.

This chapter will clear things up in layman's terms, starting with this important tip:

The primary goal of the Game is *reducing your insulin level.*

That's right, it's all about insulin, also known as the energy-storage or fat-storage hormone, because we want to *burn* energy and fat, not store it.

If you increase your insulin level, you lose the Game and win an unsightly, unhealthy sugar belly. If you do the opposite, you win the Game, flatten your belly, and transform your life. Those are your only two options.

Remember that as we review five of the most important hormones in the Game—leptin, insulin, ghrelin, dopamine, and cortisol—below.

Leptin (the "satiety hormone")

Leptin is a hormone released by your fat cells that tells your brain when you've already stored enough energy as fat, and it's time to burn some of it.

In this way, leptin naturally prevents you from overeating when it's working properly.

However, when your brain doesn't receive the leptin signal as it should, all hell breaks loose. It goes into starvation mode and directs the rest of your body to resolve the problem by reducing your energy expenditure (i.e., making you tired) and increasing your appetite (i.e., making you eat more).

Therein lies the problem with this hormone: Leptin isn't working like it used to. Something is wrong, and it's got a name: *leptin resistance*.

To visualize leptin resistance, imagine leptin trying to signal your brain that you're ready to burn some fat after a big meal, but something resists that signal, which leads your brain to think that you need another serving or, worse yet, dessert.

It's an internal communication problem with devastating consequences.

Almost all the world's 2.2 billion overweight and obese people suffer from leptin resistance, and they can't lose their sugar bellies for any significant length of time unless and until they deal with this underlying problem.

So, what's causing this resistance to the leptin signal reaching your brain?

Too much of another hormone in the Game called insulin.

And what's causing the excess insulin?

You guessed it, excessive consumption of sugar.

Insulin (The "fat storage" hormone)

Insulin is a hormone released by your pancreas that allows your body to block your leptin signal and store energy as fat for future use (weight gain).

In other words, *insulin makes sugar-belly fat.*

When your insulin level rises, your body stores more energy as fat.

When it drops, the reverse occurs. Your fat cells shrink and you lose weight.

This ebb and flow is perfectly healthy when your body is operating as a well-balanced, fat-burning machine. There are times when you want to burn energy without insulin, and other times you want to store it as fat. Storing energy as fat can be a good thing under certain circumstances.

But if you have excess insulin running through your system (also known as hyperinsulinemia), it prevents leptin from telling your brain to burn energy even when you're already stuffed. As noted above, your brain interprets (or misinterprets) this as a sign of starvation and instructs your body to (a) store more energy as fat by increasing your appetite and reducing your physical activity, and (b) release even more insulin!

Moreover, when your insulin level is too high for an extended period of time, and your fat, muscle and liver cells can't withstand the onslaught any longer, your body begins to reject or *resist* the insulin completely, creating a new set of problems in the Game.

This is called *insulin resistance*, not to be confused with leptin resistance, although both are bad for you. When it occurs in the liver, the excess sugar turns to "liver fat" and triggers production of even more insulin by the pancreas, which in turn drives even more energy storage into body fat.

Ultimately, all this excess insulin from leptin resistance and insulin resistance increases the size of your sugar belly by ensuring nonstop energy storage as fat and the weight gain that accompanies it.

It's a vicious cycle, and an all-too-common recipe for obesity.

Our insulin levels are two to four times higher today than they were 40 years ago, which is screwing up our leptin signaling, causing leptin and insulin resistance, and transforming us into a nation of sugar bellies, with the rest of the world not far behind.

Reducing Insulin and Improving Leptin Signaling

How can you break the cycle and turn the Game around?

You can reduce your insulin level and improve your leptin signaling with the Sugar Belly Secret, which is why step one involves subtracting sugar, especially sucrose (glucose and fructose) and HFCS, from your diet.

Many of the best low-carb diets recommend that you reduce your consumption of sugar and other (mostly refined or processed) foods that are high in carbohydrates that convert into sugar (glucose) in your body. If your body can't burn glucose as energy because you didn't consume many carbs, it'll burn fat for energy instead, and that's usually what happens.

These diets tend to work in the short-term because the wide net thrown over all carbs captures added sugars along with almost everything else, but most people can't or don't want to eat like this for long. There are potential health problems as well, including vitamin deficiencies, if they're not executed properly.

I tried the Ketogenic diet once and lost some weight, for example, but it made me feel sick, weak and unusually tired at times. It forced me to eliminate some non-sugary and/or high-fiber foods that I liked, too, and I'm pretty sure I caught a cold because I stopped eating fruit to reduce my daily intake of carbs.

I don't mean to knock the Ketogenic diet. It works if you stick with it, and it can be useful for dropping some pounds fast. It also includes some useful sugar-belly hacks (e.g., intermittent fasting), but I can't eat that way for more than a few days or weeks without cheating. It's just not for me.

And here's the kicker: You don't have to cut your consumption of carbs so dramatically *as long as they're low in sugar and high in fiber.*

Whole fruit contains natural sugar, for instance, but it also contains fiber that slows carbohydrate digestion and glucose absorption into the bloodstream, takes pressure off the liver, and reduces your insulin response. Plus, it's loaded with vitamins and micronutrients.

That's why the Sugar Belly Secret calls for adding fiber.

There's no need to freak out about carbs, with or without natural sugar, as long as there's enough fiber to balance things out and keep your insulin from ruining the Game.

Ghrelin (the "hunger" hormone)

While you're reducing leptin resistance and insulin resistance with the Sugar Belly Secret, there's something else you can and should reduce: your gherelin or "hunger hormone."

Reducing ghrelin will cause you to consume less food and, while the Sugar Belly Secret doesn't call for counting calories or obsessing over portion sizes, overeating is never a good idea, especially when you're trying to lose weight.

How do you reduce ghrelin?

First, make sure you're eating enough protein. Studies show that high-protein meals reduce ghrelin more than high-carb or high-fat ones. Protein-rich meals also trigger a weaker insulin response than hi-carb ones, and it's all about reducing insulin.

Second, sleep more because ghrelin increases when you're sleep deprived.

I've noticed this myself when I don't sleep enough, which is more often than I'd like to admit. I always figured that I ate more when I was sleep deprived because my body simply needed the extra energy (and lots of coffee) to wake up, but it's more than that.

It's hormonal, but we can reduce our ghrelin (decrease our appetite) by eating more protein-rich meals and getting plenty of sleep. Easy peasy.

Dopamine (The "pleasure" neurohormone)

Dopamine is a neurohormone or neurotransmitter that controls the brain's reward and pleasure centers.

According to researchers at New York University, when insulin spikes (after a tasty meal) in a normal-weight person, it triggers the release of dopamine because we love to eat—especially if the food or beverage is sugary sweet—and the dopamine generally keeps coming as long as the insulin does.

Dopamine doesn't work the same way if you're obese, however.

Studies show that obese people get the same dopamine stimulus when they see food, but they don't get the same "reward" signal after they eat it. It's just not as pleasurable as they expected it to be, presumably because the insulin is blocking this response, which make them more likely to go back for another bite… in search of that elusive reward.

I don't know exactly why this occurs, but I know that doing the same thing too many times can lead to desensitization. After a while, it's just not that great anymore. Pretty soon, we need more of it to get the same "high," or we lose interest in it altogether.

In this sense, obese people are like drug addicts. They keep going back for more of that sugary sweet stuff because they can't get enough to feel as good as they used to, and the reward for doing so becomes increasingly difficult to achieve over time.

That's a sad story about a happy hormone, but there's another hormone—arguably the most important one in your body—that you need to understand, respect and master in order to win the Game of Hormones.

Cortisol (the "stress" hormone)

We can't handle any stress in our lives without cortisol, the stress hormone.

But nobody wants too much stress, right? I certainly don't.

I've always believed that excess stress ages, weakens, and kills people faster than anything else, and as it turns out, I was right.

Excessive exposure to cortisol from stress for an extended period causes your body to generate sugar-belly fat associated with metabolic syndrome and leads to insulin resistance, sleep deprivation, and consumption of fattening "comfort foods."

What can you do about it? Plenty.

Meditate

Many health and fitness gurus recommend meditation to reduce your cortisol level, focus your mind, and help you live in the present.

If that's your thing, go for it because it works.

I practiced meditation years ago and know it helped me. I also realize that many of the world's most successful people do some form of it.

So, after a long hiatus, I'm trying it again right now, thanks to a friend who told me about an app called *Headspace*. Check it out if you're interested.

Meditation is cool and undeniably healthy, but it honestly hasn't been a big part of my stress-reduction regimen for the last 15 years.

I rely on two other things to reduce my cortisol level: Sleep and exercise.

Sleep It Off

Sleep deprivation screws up your Game by increasing cortisol, decreasing leptin, and increasing insulin, thereby significantly increasingly the likelihood of sugar belly and obesity.

Oh, and it might be killing you, too.

According to Professor Matthew Walker, director for the Centre for Human Sleep Science at the University of California, Berkeley, a "catastrophic sleep-loss epidemic" is affecting every aspect of our body chemistry and causing potentially fatal diseases and conditions, including diabetes, obesity, heart disease, Alzheimer's, stroke, and cancer.

If that ain't reason enough to get more Z's, I don't know what is.

And what could be easier than sleeping more!

You're welcome.

Walk It Off, Big Guy

You can reduce cortisol without exercise, but there's no better way to do it.

Exercise of any kind doesn't just reduce your stress level quickly, easily, and cost-effectively. It reduces your insulin resistance and burns stubborn muscle and visceral (sugar belly) fat at the same time.

You may have heard that exercise raises cortisol (stress) while you're actually doing it. That's true, but it also reduces your cortisol *for the rest of the day*.

In other words, it's totally worth it.

Plus, you'll look better if you combine exercise with the Sugar Belly Secret, especially if you'd like some more muscle to go with your slimmer waistline.

I exercise frequently now that my vertigo is gone, and I love it.

Besides improving my appearance, health and fitness, I always feel great afterwards and make new friends with similar interests. I also tend to come up with some of my best ideas in the middle of a workout. (The same thing happens in the shower, but that's neither here nor there.)

Winning!

The Sugar Belly Secret will help you to win the Game of Hormones by

- Improving your leptin signaling,
- Reducing your ghrelin,
- Keeping your dopamine working properly,
- Reducing your cortisol, and most importantly…
- Reducing your insulin level (and burning more fat)!

That's the biology of losing your sugar belly.

Now, let's take the first step of the Sugar Belly Secret by subtracting sugar.

Chapter 3 will show you exactly how to do it.

CHAPTER 3

Subtract Sugar

Back in November of 2001, when I started doing P90—the predecessor to P90X—in my home office in Miami Beach, FL, I'd take coffee breaks by walking a few blocks to Starbucks for a large ("Venti") Caffè Mocha.

Sometimes, I only drank only one a day, but most days I drank two.

I loved my Mochas and considered them a treat for all my hard work, but I couldn't help noticing something in the mirror after a while. Despite my P90 workouts, low-stress lifestyle, and fairly healthy diet (or so I thought), my belly was expanding.

I was getting fat, and I didn't know why.

Eventually, through a process of elimination (i.e., subtracting a particular food or beverage from my diet for a while to see if it made a difference), I solved the mystery.

Caffè Mocha

The culprit was my favorite thing—those Starbucks Caffè Mochas.

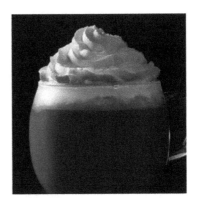

I wasn't pleased with this discovery at all, and I didn't go cold turkey right away.

I reduced my consumption to not more than one per day, but that was enough of a change to see the difference. My waistline started shrinking almost immediately.

Later, when I replaced mochas completely with regular coffee, I lost *all* of the extra weight I had been carrying. Frankly, I couldn't believe it. A relatively small change to my diet—subtracting chocolate-flavored coffee—paid off big-time.

What was it about those Caffé Mochas that made me chubby?

Starbucks answers the question right on its website.

A 20-ounce venti Caffé Mocha with whole milk and no whipped cream contains a whopping 53 grams of carbs, and *43* of them are sugar.

Venti 20oz ▼	Whole Milk ▼	No Whipped Cream ▼

Nutrition Facts Per Serving (20 fl oz)

Calories 420	Calories from Fat 140

	% Daily Value*
Total Fat 16g	25%
Saturated Fat 9g	45%
Trans Fat 0g	
Cholesterol 40mg	13%
Sodium 170mg	7%
Total Carbohydrate 53g	18%
Dietary Fiber 5g	20%
Sugars 43g	
Protein 16g	

Vitamin A 15% • Vitamin C 0% • Calcium 45% • Iron 35%

Caffeine 185mg**

*Percent Daily Values are based on a 2,000 calorie diet.

**Each caffeine value is an approximate value.

If I had added whipped cream (I didn't, but I could have), the sugar content would have risen to 45 grams, with some unhealthy trans fat thrown in for good measure.

Venti 20oz ▼	Whole Milk ▼	Whipped Cream ▼

Nutrition Facts Per Serving (20 fl oz)

Calories 490	Calories from Fat 200

	% Daily Value*
Total Fat 23g	35%
Saturated Fat 13g	65%
Trans Fat 0.5g	
Cholesterol 65mg	22%
Sodium 180mg	8%
Total Carbohydrate 55g	18%
Dietary Fiber 5g	20%
Sugars 45g	
Protein 17g	

Vitamin A 20% • Vitamin C 0% • Calcium 45% • Iron 35%

Caffeine 185mg**

*Percent Daily Values are based on a 2,000 calorie diet.

**Each caffeine value is an approximate value.

How bad is that?

A glazed donut from Dunkin' Donuts contains 12 grams of sugar, more than 3 ½ times *less* sugar than one of my Starbucks Caffé Mochas.

(To be fair, other items on the Dunkin' Donuts' menu kick sand in the face of Starbucks Caffé Mochas on sugar belly beach. If you order a Dunkin' Donuts large Vanilla Bean *Coolatta* with your glazed donut, for example, you'll add another 174 grams of sugar, increasing your total sugar rush to a sickening *186* grams.)

How about a Pepsi? According to PepsiCo's own website, a 20-ounce bottle of Pepsi contains a whopping 69 grams of sugar.

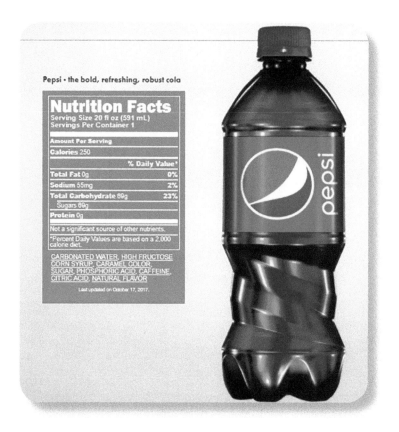

Likewise, a 20-oz. bottle of Coke clocks in at 65 grams of sugar.

My 20-oz. Caffé Mochas at Starbucks weren't as bad as a Pepsi or Coke of equal size, but they were close and, as I noted previously, I normally tossed down more than one. I was consuming 86 grams of sugar when I drank two mochas per day, and that's before considering whatever garbage I was eating with my coffee back then.

To give you a sense of how over-the-top 86 grams of sugar from two Caffè Mochas is, the World Health Organization recommends consumption of no more than 25 grams of sugar *a day*. Some U.S. government agencies allow for a higher number of grams, but here's the bottom line: The less added sugar you consume, the better, and these drinks will put you over your sugar quota for the day, all by themselves.

My inexplicably bulging sugar belly posed a problem for me back in 2001, but I identified the culprit, subtracted the sugar, lost the weight, and never looked back.

More than 15 years have passed since all that happened, and I've made plenty of nutritional mistakes since then, but drinking Caffè Mochas at Starbucks isn't one of them. I've never had another one and, honestly, I don't miss them at all. Good riddance.

Caffè Mochas were my Achilles heel.

What's *yours*?

Chances are, it's more than one food or beverage, but that's OK.

You can lose your sugar belly by spotting and subtracting sugar in the food and drinks that you consume, and the rest of this chapter will help you do it, starting with the most conspicuous troublemakers, sugar bombs.

Drop the Sugar Bombs

Do I really need to tell you to reduce your consumption of candy, cookies, cake, soda, ice cream, donuts, and other obvious sugar bombs?

Probably not, but the dazzling photos below from SinAzucar.org drive the point home with something we can all relate to, sugar cubes and blocks.

I don't mean to pick on Starbucks because I enjoy the ambiance of their cafes, and they're not alone in adding so much sugar to their products, but Starbucks' venti Frappuccino is a classic sugar bomb.

It contains 76 grams of sugar, the equivalent of 19 sugar cubes.

C'mon folks, that's gross. Drop it.

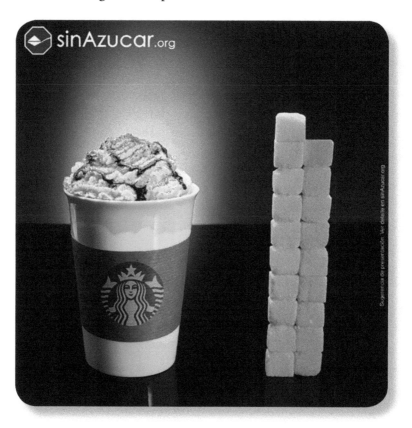

What about Cappuccino as an alternative? No harm in that, right?

While some Cappuccinos contain much less sugar than others, you're still playing with fire if you're not paying attention.

Consider Nescafe's Cappuccino, for example. More than half of it is sugar.

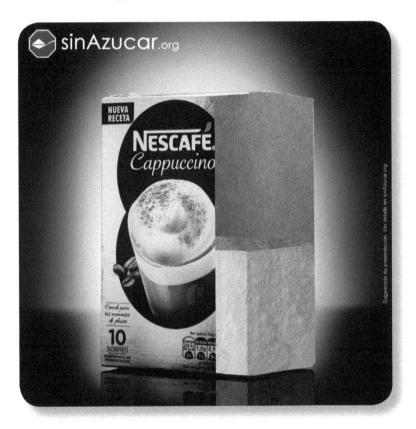

Drink regular coffee instead.

And skip the Minute Maid fruit juice while you're at it.

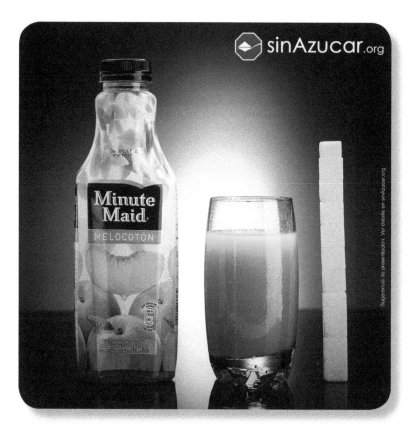

It may look healthy, but a 300 milliliter (10.14 ounce) bottle of Minute Maid Peach ("Melocoton" in Spanish) juice contains 42.9 grams of sugar. That's bad news for your belly.

Then there's Nutella.

It's delicious—I tried it a few times years ago in Germany—but it's *56.8%* sugar!

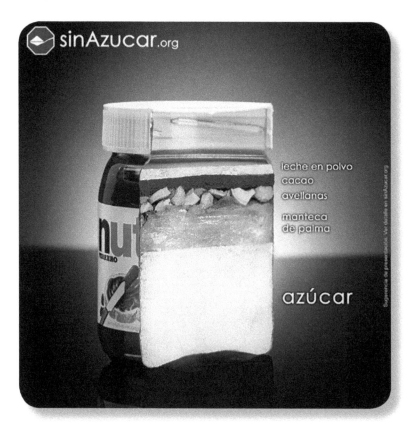

No more Nutella for you.

How about those "progressive" ice-cream boys, Ben & Jerry?

Surely, they wouldn't make people fat and sick by adding tons of sugar?

Wrong. A relatively small, 250 ml carton of Ben & Jerry's Chunky Monkey ice cream contains *60* grams of sugar, the equivalent of 15 sugar cubes.

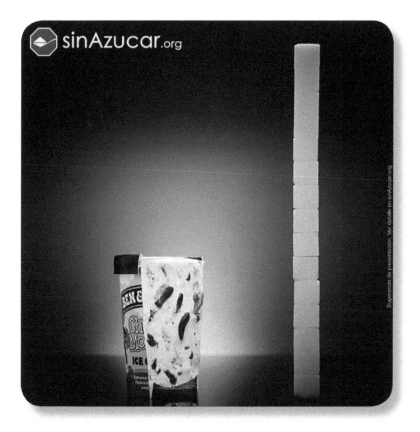

If that were a stack of poker chips, you'd be in luck, but it's not, and you're not.

Buyer beware, regardless of your political affiliation.

The same goes for energy drinks, including Red Bull, which I consumed regularly years ago by the bottle and as a mixer in my alcoholic beverages.

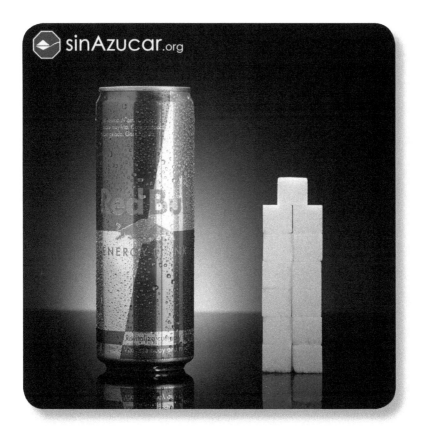

A 16-ounce bottle of Red Bull contains 52 grams of sugar.

Red Bull may or may not give you wings, but it will definitely give you a sugar belly.

So will ketchup if you're not careful.

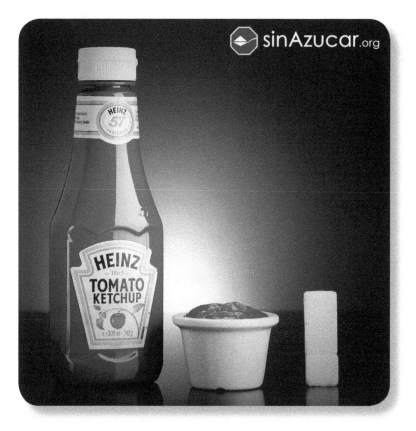

A mere 55 grams of Heinz Ketchup, for example, contain 12 grams of sugar.

It may not sound too bad after reading about huge sugar bombs like Red Bull and Nutella, but adding that much ketchup is like adding a glazed donut from Dunkin Donuts to your meal.

Will replacing Heinz Ketchup with Heinz Curry Mango Sauce solve the problem? Nope. A bottle of that stuff contains 39 grams of sugar.

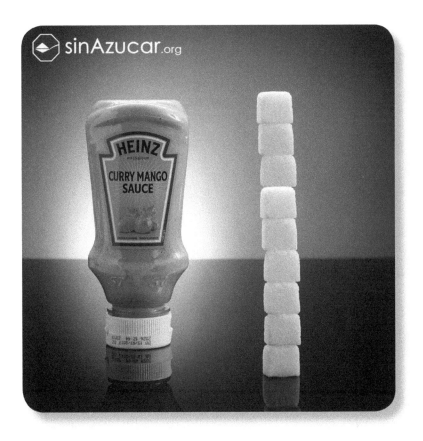

Other sugar bombs to drop from your diet immediately include:

- Mrs. Butterworth's Original Syrup (47 grams of sugar),
- Vitaminwater Focus Kiwi Strawberry (32 grams of sugar),
- Ocean Spray Cran-Apple (31 grams of sugar),
- Tazo Organic Iced Green Tea (30 grams of sugar),
- PowerBar Cookie Dough (29 grams of sugar),
- Quaker Natural Granola Apple Cranberry Almond (27 grams of sugar),
- Kashi GoLean Snacks Granola Bar (27 grams of sugar),

- Dannon All-Natural Lowfat Yogurt, Lemon (25 grams of sugar),
- KIND Almonds and Apricots Yogurt Bar (16 grams of sugar),
- Bertolli Tomato and Basil (12 grams of sugar), and
- Nature Valley Oats & Honey Granola Bars (11 grams of sugar).

I could go on, but you get the point, or at least I hope so.

Sugarspotting

Once you've dropped the sugar bombs (except for special occasions and the occasional dessert), it's time to spot and subtract much less conspicuous sugary foods and beverages from your diet.

It's tricky at times, but you can do it.

I wish I could tell you to simply check out the added sugars data on products with a Nutrition Facts label, but you won't find it on most products because the sugar lobby succeeded in pressuring the U.S. government to indefinitely delay compliance with a rule that would have required it.

In May of 2016, the Food and Drug Administration (FDA) approved a new Nutrition Facts label with a separate line for "Added Sugars" that, if implemented and enforced, would compel food and beverage companies to distinguish between natural and added sugars for the first time.

It was a smart move in my view, and they did it for the right reason. They added the new line to "*increase consumer awareness of the quantity of added sugars in foods*" (my italics) based on recommendations for reduced consumption of added sugars by organizations that really stepped up, like the American Heart Association, American Academy of Pediatrics, Institute of Medicine, and the World Health Organization.

Here's a side-by-side comparison of the old label with the new one:

Old Label:

Nutrition Facts

Serving Size 2/3 cup (55g)
Servings Per Container About 8

Amount Per Serving

Calories 230	Calories from Fat 72

	% Daily Value*
Total Fat 8g	12%
Saturated Fat 1g	5%
Trans Fat 0g	
Cholesterol 0mg	0%
Sodium 160mg	7%
Total Carbohydrate 37g	12%
Dietary Fiber 4g	16%
Sugars 1g	
Protein 3g	

Vitamin A	10%
Vitamin C	8%
Calcium	20%
Iron	45%

* Percent Daily Values are based on a 2,000 calorie diet. Your daily value may be higher or lower depending on your calorie needs.

	Calories:	2,000	2,500
Total Fat	Less than	65g	80g
Sat Fat	Less than	20g	25g
Cholesterol	Less than	300mg	300mg
Sodium	Less than	2,400mg	2,400mg
Total Carbohydrate		300g	375g
Dietary Fiber		25g	30g

New Label:

Nutrition Facts

8 servings per container
Serving size   2/3 cup (55g)

Amount per serving

Calories   230

	% Daily Value*
Total Fat 8g	10%
Saturated Fat 1g	5%
Trans Fat 0g	
Cholesterol 0mg	0%
Sodium 160mg	7%
Total Carbohydrate 37g	13%
Dietary Fiber 4g	14%
Total Sugars 12g	
Includes 10g Added Sugars	20%
Protein 3g	

Vitamin D 2mcg	10%
Calcium 260mg	20%
Iron 8mg	45%
Potassium 235mg	6%

* The % Daily Value (DV) tells you how much a nutrient in a serving of food contributes to a daily diet. 2,000 calories a day is used for general nutrition advice.

As you can see, the new label includes a larger, more realistic description of "Serving size" and "servings per container," but best part is the new "Added Sugars" information.

The new label would make sugarspotting significantly easier precisely when many people need it most, but it does have a few deficiencies.

Most importantly, the FDA carved out a "juice" loophole by defining Added Sugars to exclude "fruit and vegetable juice concentrated from 100% fruit juice … as well as some sugars found in fruit and vegetable juices, jellies, jams, preserves, and fruit spreads." There's technically no added sugar in juice, but many leading experts claim that the sugar in juice equates to added sugar as soon as companies that make it extract the fiber from the fruit and vegetables during processing, and I believe them.

What exactly happened to the FDA's new Nutrition Facts label?

When the FDA announced its new rule in May of 2016, it set a compliance date of July 26, 2018, with an extra year to comply for manufacturers with annual food sales of less than $10 million. Allowing companies sufficient time to change their labeling made sense, but it also opened a window of opportunity for the sugar lobby to pressure government officials to delay or scuttle the whole thing, and that's what they did.

On June 13, 2017, after "industry and consumer groups provided the FDA with feedback regarding the compliance dates," the FDA announced its intention to extend the compliance dates... *indefinitely.*

Boom.

Some large food and beverage companies modified their Nutrition Facts labels anyway, for one reason or another. Early adopters include Nabisco/ Mondelez, which put the labels on its Wheat Thins crackers; KIND, which applied them on its granola bars; and believe it or not, PepsiCo, which pasted them on its Lay's chips, Fritos and Cheetos.

Those companies deserve credit for being responsible and simplifying our sugarspotting, but others used the "juice" loophole in the new Nutrition Facts label to make their products seem healthier than they actually are.

Naked Juice, Inc., a California-based producer of juices and smoothies, for example, modified their label to show "Incl. 0g Added Sugars" under "Total Sugars 53g." Don't be fooled by this kind of deceptive labeling.

If natural sugar from juice is just as fattening as added sugar because the fiber has been removed from the fruits and vegetables during processing, then this is just a sneaky way of making this product seem healthy, persuading you to drink it, and making you fat.

Incidentally, I used to drink Naked Juice's "Green Machine" regularly years ago when I was getting soft and fat. It tastes great and certainly looks healthy at first glance, but I either never guessed that it contains 53 grams of sugar or didn't bother to look, and I didn't understand the importance of fiber back then.

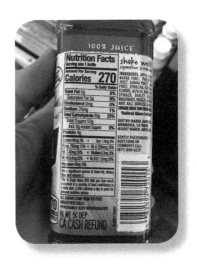

Well, I don't make that mistake anymore and doubt I'll ever drink another bottle of Naked Juice for the rest of my life.

I eat real, whole fruit and vegetables instead, and so should you.

Fortunately, perhaps because so many multinational corporations voluntarily adopted the new Nutrition Facts label, or because of pressure from consumers who started expecting to see it on new products and insisting that companies fess up, or maybe just because government officials realized that they couldn't justify an indefinite delay in the new labeling regulations any longer, the FDA has finally imposed a new deadline.

On September 29, 2017, the FDA announced that large companies will have until January 1, 2020 to comply with the new regulations and start printing the new Nutrition Facts labels on all their processed and packaged products. Smaller companies have another year, until January 1, 2021, to implement the same changes.

That's good if not great news (better late than never), but your sugar belly, health, and fitness can't wait until the next decade to start making smarter, more informed decisions as a consumer, and neither can mine.

We need to start fighting back by working with the nutritional information and tools at our disposal today, and we've got some pretty good ones.

Besides taking the "Total Sugars" data on existing Nutrition Facts labels into account—if the Total Sugars in a product is high, *forget it*—keep a close eye on ingredients lists because food and beverage companies use them to surreptitiously add sugar by calling it something else.

The list of alternative names for processed or added sugar, which you should learn to spot on ingredients labels, includes the following:

- Agave (juice/nectar/sap/ syrup)
- Baker's sugar
- Bar sugar
- Barbados sugar
- Beet sugar
- Blackstrap molasses
- Brown (sugar/rice syrup)
- Buttered syrup
- Cane (juice/sugar/syrup/ crystals)
- Caramel
- Carob (syrup/powder)
- Castor sugar (aka Berry sugar)
- Chinese Rock Sugar
- Clintose
- Confectioner's (powdered) sugar
- Corn (syrup/glucose syrup/ sweetener)
- Crystalline fructose
- Date sugar
- Demerara sugar
- Dextrose
- Drimol
- Drisweet
- Dried raisin sweetener
- Edible lactose
- Evaporated cane juice
- Flomalt
- Florida crystals
- Fructose (sweetener)
- Fruit juice (concentrate)
- Gemsugar
- Glazed and icing sugar
- Glaze icing sugar
- Golden (sugar/syrup)
- Gomme
- Grape (sugar/syrup)
- Granular sweetener
- Granulated sugar
- High-fructose corn syrup
- Honey
- Honibake

- Honiflake
- Icing sugar
- Invert sugar (aka Trimoline)
- Isoglucose
- Isomaltulose
- Kona ame
- Lactose
- Liquid sweetener
- Malt
- Maltose
- Maple (sugar/syrup)
- Mizu ame
- Molasses
- Muscovado sugar
- Nulomoline
- Organic raw sugar
- Panella (aka Rapadura)
- Panoche
- Powdered sugar
- Raw sugar
- Refiner's sugar
- Rice syrup
- Rock sugar
- Sorghum (syrup)
- Starch sweetener
- Sucanat
- Sucrose
- Sucrovert
- Sugar beet
- Sugar invert
- Sweet n neat
- Table sugar
- Treacle
- Trehalose
- Tru sweet
- Turbinado sugar
- Vanilla sugar
- Versatose, and
- Wasanbon
- Yellow sugar

The more familiar you are with these code names for sugar, the more likely you are to avoid products that contain them when food and beverage companies try to pull a fast one.

Subtract, Subtract, Subtract

A recent study demonstrated that the major sources of sugar in the American diet are as follows:

- Sugar-sweetened beverages (37.1%),
- Sweet baked goods like cakes, cookies and donuts (13.7%),
- Fruit juice drinks (8.9%),
- Dairy desserts like ice cream (6.1%), and
- Candy (5.8%).

Your mission is to subtract as much of this stuff from your diet as possible.

What's the best way to do it?

Listen up.

Subtract All Beverages Except Water and Milk

Start by trashing any and all sugared beverages that you've already purchased, including soda, juice, energy drinks, and vitamin water.

You can keep unsweetened milk because it contains lactose, a relatively harmless and not particularly sweet type of sugar that your body converts into glucose, not fructose, as well as many important vitamins and micronutrients.

But everything else must go.

That includes fruit juice because *juice normally has more teaspoons of sugar per cup than soda.*

So, don't drink your fruit; eat it whole… with the fiber intact.

When you're done cleaning house, the only beverages left should be water and milk, but unsweetened coffee and tea are perfectly fine. (I drink a few cups of black coffee almost every day).

As for sugar-free sodas and other sugar-free or "lite" products, you can consume them in moderation as an alternative to sugary ones if you must—I cheat with Stevia in some of my snack foods, for example—but you're better off trashing them too for three reasons.

First, according to an August 2017 study by researchers at Yale University, sugar-free, low-calorie and other "diet" drinks and foods trick your brain into making you fatter. This occurs because your brain associates the taste of something sweet with an infusion of sugar and energy and acts accordingly by signaling your pancreas to create more insulin, which makes you fat.

Scientists aren't sure exactly what happens when you're brain finally realizes that the sugar and energy didn't arrive on cue, but many believe that this sleight of hand in the Game of Hormones makes you crave sugar elsewhere, and that craving causes problems.

Professor Dana Small, who authored the study, put it this way: "A calorie is not a calorie." That is, "[w]hen sweet taste and energy [from sugar and carb calories] are not matched, less energy is metabolized and inaccurate signals go to the brain. Either may affect metabolic health."

Second, and this point is undoubtedly related to the first, artificial sweeteners cause sugar belly, too. A 2015 study by the *Journal of the American Geriatrics Society* found a link between increased consumption of diet sodas and abdominal obesity. More specifically, the study found that older adults who drank diet soda daily saw their waist size increase over 3X more than those who didn't over a period of nine years.

Third, the jury is still out on how all these new artificial sweeteners affect your health and fitness in the long-term. Who knows what they really do? It's a crap shoot.

In light of all that, why take the chance?

Most sugar-free stuff tastes like chemicals anyway, and you won't miss it after a while. You may even notice that, once you stop drinking diet sodas and beverages, you'll lose your craving for it completely and wonder why you ever drank it in the first place.

Subtract Foods That Don't Pass the Test

Got donuts, cake, or cookies at home?

Bad reader. All of that belongs in the trash can.

Please move it there, right now, and give yourself some credit for doing so.

Then do the same thing with all other food in your refrigerator and cabinets that can't pass the sugar-belly test.

To pass the sugar-belly test, a food product must contain:

1) Little or no added sugar,
   o Caveat: You don't have to throw away every food product with some added sugar (that's not realistic or sustainable) but use your head. If it contains more grams of added sugar than fiber, toss it.
2) At least 3 grams of fiber, and
3) No trans fat or Omega-6 fats.
   o Caveat: Most "fats" are healthy and delicious—I love my avocado and nuts, for example—but foods containing harmful processed trans fat or Omega-6 fats should be removed from your shopping list permanently.

If you need a bigger trash can after this subtraction exercise, you're probably doing it right. Everything that fails the test must go.

As for all that new empty space in your fridge and kitchen cabinets, don't worry. Nature abhors a vacuum. Before you know it, you'll be buying real, healthy food to eat at home instead, and your sugar belly will vanish along with the stuff that created it.

Dine Out Wisely

I'm a bachelor who doesn't cook or keep a lot of food or beverages in my house. I don't enjoy cooking for one and overeat if I have food around while I'm working at home.

That means I dine out several times every day, and I've gotten good at it.

I screw up occasionally when I go to a new restaurant and am unfamiliar with the menu, but I've learned how to order food and drinks that are low in added sugar and high in fiber most of the time, and I eat really well.

Restaurant food is tricky because it's normally served with little or no nutritional information. It may look great on the menu, but appearances can be deceiving.

Here are some facts about added sugar in foods from some of America's most popular restaurants to illustrate the point, all of which is easily accessible online:

Applebee's:

- Pecan-Crusted Chicken Salad (65 grams of sugar)
- 4-Cheese Mac & Cheese with Honey Pepper Chicken Tenders (53 grams of sugar)

California Pizza Kitchen:

- Pork Chop Chop Salad (68 grams of sugar)
- Thai Crunch Salad (51 grams of sugar)

Cheesecake Factory:

- French Toast Napoleon with Syrup (139 grams of sugar)
- Bruleed French Toast (120 grams of sugar)

Chili's:

- Crispy Honey Chipotle & Waffles (105 grams of sugar)
- Caribbean Salad with Grilled Chicken (70 grams of sugar)
- Crispy Fiery Pepper (55 grams of sugar)
- Boneless Wings, Honey Chipotle (40 grams of sugar)

IHOP:

- Banana Crepes with Nutella (67 grams of sugar)
- Cinn-A-Stacks Pancakes (60 grams of sugar)

Longhorn Steakhouse:

- Grilled Chicken and Strawberry Salad (41 grams of sugar)
- Churrasco Steak with Plantains (31 grams of sugar)
- Kids Fountain Drink (312 grams of sugar!)

P.F. Chang's:

- Spicy Chicken, Gluten-free (90 grams of sugar)
- Sweet and Sour Chicken (69 grams of sugar)
- Beef a la Sichuan (67 grams of sugar)

Yardhouse:

- Nashville Hot Chicken (75 grams of sugar)
- Maui Pineapple Chicken (73 grams of sugar)
- Sweet Potato Fries (42 grams of sugar)

How can you reduce the likelihood of consuming too much sugar when you dine out?

Here are a few rules of thumb that have served me well:

- Tell your server that you don't want any bread, chips, or croutons in the food or on the table, even if you're ordering a hamburger with bacon. Just tell him or her that you don't eat those things, so they might as well save them for someone else.

- Skip dessert, except for special occasions. Most dessert items in restaurants have added sugar up the wazoo. I know this doesn't sound like fun, but you'll be surprised how easy it is to say "No" to dessert after a while. You'll simply stop craving them in the same way.

- If you're thinking of buying a food or beverage that comes in a package, bottle or wrapper, read the Nutrition Facts label, and pay special attention to the amount of Total Sugars and fiber, as well as the serving size. If it doesn't score well, don't buy it.

- Many salad dressings contain added sugar that can turn your healthy salad into an insulin rush. Stick to ones with 0 to 2 grams of sugar.

- Avoid fast food, which is typically sugary, fiberless, and unhealthy, *unless* you've viewed their nutritional menu (online) and found something that's relatively low in sugar and high in fiber, with no trans fat. It'll take a few minutes to investigate, but you can usually find an item or two that won't make your sugar belly worse than it is.

- Drink regular coffee most of the time. You can add milk if you like—I do it, and my biggest weakness right now is cappuccinos because I know there's some lactose in there—but stay away from the fancy, sugar-rich coffee drinks at cafes and elsewhere.

- Drink unsweetened water, not soda, juice or alcohol (except red wine in moderation).

- Order food loaded with healthy proteins (e.g., baked or grilled chicken, turkey, steak, eggs), fats (e.g., avocado, bacon, nuts, seeds), and carbs (vegetables, fruits and other stuff that's high in fiber and relatively low in added sugar, like *Fiber One* cereal).

- Lastly, don't make too many assumptions or take too many chances. Get the facts before you consume something. If you suspect that a particular dish may be high in sugar, either don't order it or quickly Google it to find out what's up. You can almost always find enough nutritional information online to make a well-informed decision about what you plan to eat or drink.

Step one for losing your sugar belly involves subtracting as much sugar from your diet as possible. I realize that giving up something you like can be a drag, and we all love the taste of sugar, but help is on the way.

Step two of the Sugar Belly Secret eases the pain and makes the entire weight-loss program extraordinarily sustainable because you get to *add* delicious foods that are off-limits in carb-Nazi diets, *as long as they're high in fiber.*

Chapter four will show you how to do it.

CHAPTER 4

Add Fiber

I used to think only old, constipated people needed fiber, but I was wrong.

It's your secret weapon in the war on sugar belly.

Fiber not only helps to prevent sugar belly; it also allows you eat a lot tastier carbs than you would otherwise be able to consume without getting fat.

Many high-carb diets work precisely because fiber mitigates the impact of the extra carbs.

However, like a good man or woman, fiber is increasingly hard to find.

Food companies have removed all or most of the fiber from many foods because it reduces shelf life, extends the time required to cook and eat the food, and makes products more expensive, none of which is helpful to a multinational industry trying to maximize profits and market share.

Consequently, we end up eating food with little or no fiber and too much sugar, which is exactly why the first two steps of a sugar belly breakthrough are countermeasures—subtract the added sugar and add the fiber.

It's simple, really, but you've got to stay alert and modify your consumption habits if you're going to *un-process* your diet… and keep it real.

I experienced this recently on trips to two of the biggest grocery stores in Medellin, Colombia, where I am as I write this. Each time, I went in search of my favorite high-fiber cereal, *Fiber One* (14 grams of fiber, 0 grams of sugar) and didn't find it. I tried to find a similar, possibly

Colombian alternative, but nothing came close. Every Nutrition Facts label I examined was high in added sugar and/or relatively low in fiber.

The best I could get was *All Bran* (12 grams of fiber, 9 grams of sugar). It's OK for occasional consumption because the fiber count is so high, but I tend to overeat cereal when it tastes like a snack, and *All Bran* is surprisingly sweet. So, I went home empty-handed.

No worries. I stopped eating as much cereal here in Colombia—at least until I find a great one—and replaced it with other breakfast foods that are higher in fiber. It really wasn't hard to do either, even here in Medellin.

Why is it important to find, buy and eat at least some foods that are high in fiber? Because fiber belly helps prevent sugar belly.

That's right, fiber is your friend and ally in the battle against sugar belly. It can help you win the Game of Hormones... if you put it in play.

Fiber Belly

Fiber protects us from sugar by acting like a traffic cop in our intestines.

Without getting overly technical and boring you to tears, it works like this:

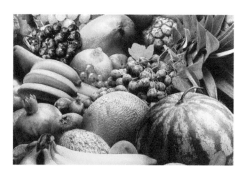

There are two types of healthy fiber, soluble and insoluble.

Most plant-based foods and fruit contain some combination of soluble and insoluble fiber. When you eat a fibrous food, the fiber races to your intestines and sets up a temporary roadblock for sugar and other carbs.

Insoluble fiber serves as the principle barrier because it's harder, and soluble fiber (which turns into a gel-like substance in the stomach) plugs gaps within it.

Then they team up to do three things.

First, the soluble and insoluble fiber redirect some of the energy (sugar and other carbs) from our food to intestinal bacteria that eat it, thereby reducing carb absorption into the rest of your body, while letting vitamins and micronutrients pass through unimpeded.

Second, when these fibrous traffic cops release other energy into our bloodstream, they do so at a far slower rate (making sure it observes the lower speed limit), which protects our liver, pancreas, and brain from a sugar rush that would flood the body with excess, fat-producing insulin.

Third, fiber also helps our brains receive the leptin ("satiety") signal sooner because it reaches the end of the intestine faster than everything else, makes us feel full (satiated), and diminishes our craving for another serving.

In short, fiber limits our absorption of fructose (which otherwise screws with the liver) and other potentially fattening carbs, reduces our insulin response, and improves leptin signaling, all of which prevents sugar belly.

In other words, fiber is surprisingly cool.

That's why the *quality* of our calories matters as much or more than the quantity, and why calorie counting as a weight loss strategy often fails.

When you eat fruit, vegetables, and unprocessed complex carbs high in fiber, your intestinal bacteria dispense with many of those calories before they're released into your bloodstream and slow down the rest in a way that makes them less likely to produce sugar belly.

Not too shabby, huh?

What about fruit juice?

Appearances can be deceiving.

Fruit juice tricks most people, including me for many years, because it *seems* healthy. Who could object to a glass of orange juice?!? But it's a Trojan horse for sugar.

Juices and smoothies actually *cause* sugar belly because companies remove all or almost all the fiber from the fruit during processing.

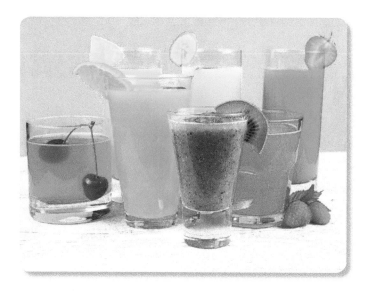

Without a fibrous checkpoint to redirect some of that sugar to your ravenous intestinal bacteria and slow down the rest, juice unleashes mayhem on your metabolism and contributes mightily to sugar belly.

Don't drink your fruit. Eat real, fibrous, whole fruit, instead.

Fiberspotting

Losing a sugar belly requires some advanced fiberspotting skills, but it's much easier than sugarspotting if you remember to do a few simple things.

First, when your read Nutrition Facts labels, check to see how many grams of fiber the food contains, and how much of it is soluble and insoluble. Food companies can't hide the ball like they do with "Added Sugar." They're required to disclose the amount and type of fiber in their labeled products, but it's up to you to notice and read all about it.

If a food product contains at least as many grams of fiber as added sugar, it won't hurt you. Otherwise, keep looking.

Second, if a food or beverage doesn't include a Nutrition Facts label and you're not sure about the grams of fiber and added sugar it contains, search for information about it online. Often, you'll quickly find the answers you need.

Third, if you're in a restaurant and can't rely on a Nutrition Facts label or internet search for nutritional information, use your head. Take some time to learn about which foods provide some fiber to offset the (sugary) carbs that you're consuming, and which ones don't. Then order the good stuff.

Spot and Avoid This

Fruit juices and smoothies

Just say no to fruit juices and smoothies unless you want a sugar belly.

That goes for prune juice, too. Unlike most fruit juice, prune juice contains a few grams of fiber, but it also contains way too much added sugar to make it worthwhile. Eat prunes, instead. Problem solved.

White foods

From now on, pass on the white foods, especially white rice, pasta, bread, and pancakes and waffles made from white refined flour.

So much for white privilege.

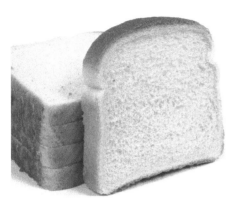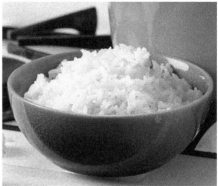

White foods need to go because they tend to be synonymous with processed, low-fiber ones that cause and exacerbate sugar belly.

The only possible exception to the general rule relates to white potatoes if you consume the skin as well. I rarely eat them because they're so high in starchy carbs and sugar (4.2 grams per potato), but they do offer a lot of fiber (8.9 grams) and some protein (6.2 grams) to balance things out.

Sugary, low-fiber cereals

The majority of cold cereals contribute to sugar belly because they don't contain nearly enough fiber to match all of the added sugar.

There are too many losers to mention, but some of the worst offenders are:

- Quaker Oat's Cap'n Crunch – 15.69 grams of sugar and 0.9 grams of fiber per cup,

- Kellogg's Honey Smacks – 15 grams of sugar and 1 gram of fiber per cup,

- Post's Golden Crisp Cereal – 14 grams of sugar and 1 gram of fiber per cup,

- Kellogg's Smorz – 13 grams of sugar and 1 gram of fiber per cup,

- General Mill's Lucky Charms – 12.6 grams of sugar and 1.8 grams of fiber,
- Kellogg's Apple Jacks with Marshmallows – 12 grams of sugar and 2 grams of fiber per cup, and
- Quaker Oat's Honey Graham Oh's Cereal – 12 grams of sugar and 1 gram of fiber per cup.

Still not ready to stop eating this stuff?

Consider this: A box of every one of the cereals above contains over 40% sugar (visualize the sugar cubes), and a few contain over 50% sugar, with Kellogg's Honey Smacks topping the list at 56.6% sugar… and just 1 gram of fiber.

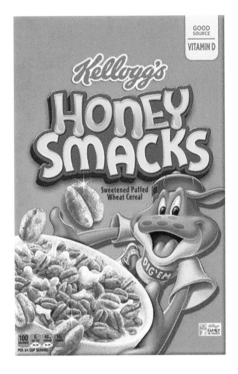

C'mon. Don't smack your nutrition upside the head by eating a box of sugar.

By way of comparison, a Hostess Twinkie contains 16 grams of sugar and no fiber. The cereals on my list above are slightly better than that if all you eat is one cup, but who stops at just one cup of cereal in the morning?

Most fast food

Most fast food is low in fiber and high in added sugar—the recipe for sugar belly—and should be avoided wherever and whenever possible.

McDonalds Hotcakes, for example, contain 45 grams of sugar and just 2 grams of fiber. They will make you fat, with or without the syrup and butter.

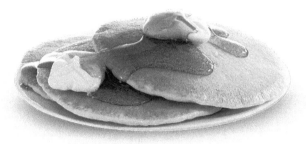

I could provide a thousand more examples of fast food that causes sugar belly, but think of it this way: When in doubt about fast food, don't eat it. Assume the worst, and you'll usually be right. You're better off going hungry for a while until you find some real food.

However, let's be fair. If you do your sugar-belly research, you can usually find a least one item on any fast-food menu that isn't a nutritional disaster, and a few that aren't bad at all.

McDonald's Bacon Ranch Salad with Buttermilk Crispy Chicken, for example, contains 4 grams of fiber, 4 grams of sugar, and 33 grams of protein. I'm not sure how it tastes, but if I had to eat at McDonalds, I'd order one of these with water or unsweetened coffee.

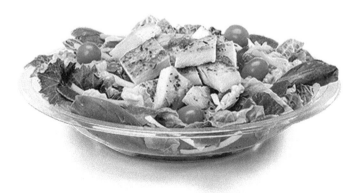

McDonald's classic Egg McMuffin ain't bad, either. It contains 2 grams of fiber, 3 grams of sugar, and 18 grams of protein. I ordered one last week on my way to an event and didn't feel at all guilty about scarfing it down.

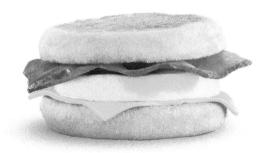

Spot and Eat This

There are many ways to add fiber for a sugar-belly breakthrough, depending on the type of food you enjoy eating each day.

Just pick and choose from the list below, or find other high-fiber, low-sugar foods to ensure that you're consuming your carbs with fiber from one source or another.

Vegetables

Look, I'm not going to pretend to be one of those guys who loves veggies, but some taste better than others, and I eat them almost every day because they provide important micronutrients and sugar-belly fighting fiber.

Some notably good sources of fiber include:

- *Artichokes* – More fiber per serving than any other vegetable,
- *Green peas* – 8.8 grams of fiber per cup when boiled,
- *Parsnip* (not to be confused with catnip)– 7 grams of fiber per cup when cooked,

- *Broccoli* – 5.1 grams of fiber per cup when boiled,
- *Brussels sprouts* – 4.1 grams of fiber per cup when boiled,
- *Spinach* – 4 grams of fiber per cup when cooked,
- *Sweet corn* – 3.6 grams of fiber per cup when boiled, and
- *Carrots* – 2.3 grams of fiber per half-cup when cooked.

Fruits

I love whole fruit as a source of fiber, despite the natural sugar that accompanies it. I consider it a dessert and rarely overdo it, but the ability to eat fruit and still lose my sugar belly is pretty awesome.

Some all-stars in the fruit category include:

- *Raspberries* – 8 grams of fiber per cup, raw,
- *Blackberries* – 7.6 grams of fiber per cup, raw,
- *Avocado* – This superfood, which I used to shun but now love, contains 6.7 grams of fiber per cup, raw. It's also full of vitamins and healthy fats,
- *Pears* – 5.5 grams of fiber, with the skin,
- *Apples* – 4.4 grams of fiber, with the skin,
- *Bananas and Oranges* – 3.1 grams of fiber, medium-sized, and
- *Strawberries* – 3.0 grams of fiber per cup.

Legumes, Seeds and Nuts

This group of foods offers a powerful punch of fiber and more. If you're not eating at least some of them regularly already, now's the time to start.

- *Split peas* – 16.3 grams of fiber per cup when boiled, and protein-rich,
- *Lentils* – 15.6 grams of fiber per cup when boiled,

- *Black beans* – 15 grams of fiber per cup when cooked, loaded with protein and complex carbs, and—unlike sugary sweet baked beans—extremely low in sugar,

- *Chia seeds* – This is one of the healthiest foods you can eat. It packs 11 grams of fiber, 4 grams of protein, 9 grams of healthy fat, and all sorts of vitamins and antioxidants, in every 1 ounce (about 2 tablespoons) serving … and they have a mild, nutty flavor that makes it easy to add them to almost anything.

- *Lima beans* – 9 grams of fiber per cup, cooked or canned,

- *Whole Quinoa* – This superfood is often categorized as a whole grain, but it's technically a seed, so I put it here to make seed-eating cooler. It contains 5 grams of fiber and 0 grams of sugar when cooked.

QUINOA

Nutrition Facts

serving size: 1 cup, cooked

calories	222
total fat	4 g
total carbs	39 g
dietary fiber	5 g
sugars	0 g
protein	8 g

vitamins & minerals

vitamin E	6%
thiamin	13%
iron	15%
magnesium	30%
phosphorus	28%
zinc	13%
copper	18%
manganese	58%

simplyquinoa.com

- *Amaranth* – This is another seed, like quinoa, with grain-like qualities. It contains 5.2 grams of fiber per cup.

- *Almonds* – 3.5 grams of fiber per ounce (23 nuts),

- *Pistachio nuts* – 2.9 grams of fiber per ounce (49 nuts), and

- *Pecans* – 2.7 grams of fiber per ounce (19 halves).

High-Fiber, Low-Sugar Bran Cereal

You can add fiber to your diet by eating bran cereal… if you choose wisely.

My two favorites are:

- *Shredded Wheat,* no added sugar – 6 grams of fiber and 0 grams of sugar per serving, and

- *Fiber One* – 14 grams of fiber and 0 grams of sugar, per serving.

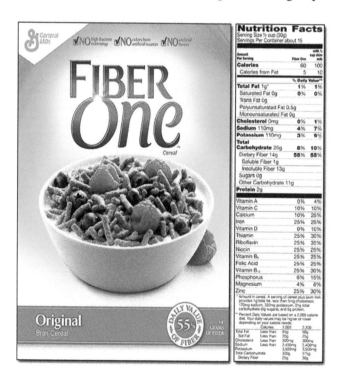

High-fiber, Whole-grain Bread

You can eat bread too, if you get it from a high-fiber, low-added-sugar loaf, but be careful here.

Please don't assume that a bread or grain product is high in fiber and low in sugar just because you see the word "wheat." Most companies who make wheat bread add sugar and coloring to make it look healthier (and less processed) than it actually is. Beware of bread products with the words "light" or even "high fiber." Check the label before you buy!

For example, here's a "Fit Integral" loaf of bread from a company named *Bimbo* that I bought recently in Medellin, Colombia, hoping it would rise above its name.

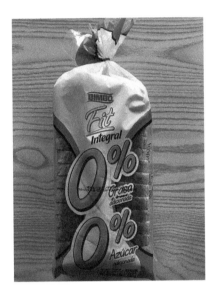

As you can see, they plastered "0% Added Sugar" (in Spanish) right on the front of the packaging. Intrigued, I flipped it over to check out the Nutrition Facts label and, while it does contain 2 grams of sugar per serving (2 slices), it also contains 4 grams of fiber and 10 grams of healthy protein. Not bad!

I'm sure you can find bread with less sugar and more fiber than mine in the United States or wherever you are when you read this. Whole Foods and Trader Joes probably offer better options, but I can eat a couple of slices of Bimbo bread every once in a while without worrying about sugar belly.

Other unsweetened whole grains

- *Pearled barley* – Eat pearled barley (6 grams of fiber when cooked) instead of foolishly trying to drink it in beer (0 grams of fiber),

- *Oatmeal* – 4 grams of fiber when cooked, and

- *Brown or wild rice:* Go with long-grain brown rice (1.8 grams of fiber per half cup when cooked) or wild rice instead of the white stuff.

High-Fiber, Low-Sugar Treats

Some treats strike an acceptable balance between fiber and sugar and can be consumed in moderation. For example:

- *Air-popped popcorn* – Some popcorn is bad for you—buttered movie theatre popcorn contains up to 4.5 grams of harmful trans fat, for example—but 3 cups of air-popped popcorn contain almost no sugar (0.2 grams), no trans fat, and 3.6 grams of fiber.

- *Quest (Cookies and Cream) Protein Bar* – As a rule, you should avoid protein bars because they're highly processed and the contents are hard to decipher, but I confess to eating Quest protein bars every now and then. My favorite is the Cookies and Cream, which contains 14 grams of fiber, 1 gram of sugar, and 21 grams of protein.

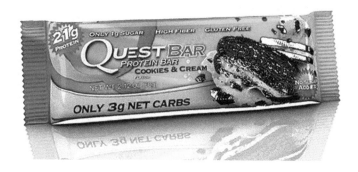

- *Other Treats that Pass the Sugar Belly Test* – If you read nutrition labels and ingredient lists carefully, you can find other treats that are high in fiber and low in sugar. I just returned from a trip to a health food store here in Medellin and came home with a few bags of my favorite *Elemental* protein cookies, for example. They have various kinds, but my favorite is the Coconut Orange, which contains 21.6 grams of protein, no sugar, and 10 grams of fiber. They've added some Stevia, but it appears dead last on the ingredient list. That works for me.

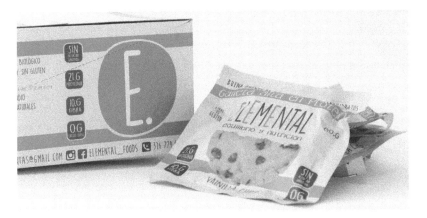

Tough Calls

- *Whole Wheat Pasta* – Think *all* pasta is off limits because of the carb content? Nope. If you choose the right whole-wheat pasta (6.3 grams of fiber when cooked), and the sugar level isn't off the charts, you may be good to go. Just remember to check the label very carefully.

- *Sweet Potatoes, with the Skin:* Everyone raves about sweet potatoes, and it's true that they contain lots of vitamins and micronutrients, but a single 130-gram sweet potato contains 5.43 grams of sugar and only 3.9 grams of fiber. The fiber is good, but that's a lot of sugar. Think twice before throwing down one of these if there are other options.

Is there any downside to adding fiber in step two of the Sugar Belly Secret?

Yeah, but it's no big deal.

If you add *too much* fiber to your diet, it can cause temporary bloating, intestinal discomfort, and way too many trips to the bathroom hours later.

So, start by adding a little more each day and see how your body responds, rather than hitting it with half a box of *Fiber One*.

In addition, even if you add just the right amount of fiber to your diet, you should expect more, ahem, flatulence.

That's right. You're going to increase your carbon footprint by emitting a bit more gas into the atmosphere, just like the cows.

But look at the bright side…

You'll be literally farting your sugar belly away.

Just don't overdo it, for your sake… and mine.

CHAPTER 5

Subtract Alcohol

My old buddy, fitness guru Tony Horton, didn't drink alcohol back in the early P90X days, or at least that's what he said. I remember attending a party to celebrate completion of the P90X test group with the whole gang. Everyone was drinking beer or cocktails, except Tony who, to his credit, didn't need it to have a good time.

Legendary boxer Floyd Mayweather allegedly doesn't drink alcohol either, even though he owns a strip club in Las Vegas and attends regularly.

Does that mean you need to stop drinking alcohol completely to lose your sugar belly?

Absolutely not.

I certainly won't quit because I enjoy drinking socially, like most people.

My go-to drink is red wine because, as explained more fully below, it contains valuable antioxidants and may actually *prevent* sugar belly if consumed in moderation.

I also find that soda water with lime quenches my thirst, serves as a great substitute for alcohol, and actually *looks* like a real drink, which reduces peer pressure to indulge.

But I'm not gonna lie. I consume other types of alcohol besides red wine occasionally, too. I rarely drink excessively, but I've been known to get a buzz on special occasions.

A few months ago, for example, I was invited to big concert in Medellin, Colombia with a group of 6 guys from my dance school, most of whom I didn't know very well. They were all drinking cheap Colombian beer, and one of the guys was buying for everyone. I thought about declining and drinking bottled water instead, but I couldn't do it. It was a rare opportunity to bond with new friends with similar interests in a foreign country, and I didn't want to be a party pooper or the odd-man out.

The next day, I felt guilty about it, but I didn't let it ruin my day. I got right back on the sugar-belly wagon and stayed there.

Nobody's perfect, and any weight-loss system that requires perfection is unrealistic and unsustainable for almost all of us.

Drink Smarter

If you already don't drink alcohol for any reason, you're ahead of the game. You can skip this chapter and move to the next one if you wish.

But if you're like me and enjoy drinking socially, you don't have to go cold turkey to lose your sugar belly. You just have to drink smarter.

Believe it or not, a daily ration of alcohol can actually help to prevent obesity and metabolic syndrome, especially if your drink of choice is red wine, but it's gotta be *small*.

The problem rests with excess consumption of alcoholic drinks. Drinking heavily inevitably leads to sugar belly (or beer belly) and metabolic syndrome, even if you're crushing it in step one and two of this system.

Far too many people are drinking excessively these days, and it shows.

According to two large national surveys, the number of people who received a diagnosis of alcoholism between 2001-2002 and 2012-2013 increased more than 49% in the United States, affecting 12.7% of the total population.

That means *more than 1 in 8 Americans now qualify as alcoholics.*

Nobody wants to give up their alcohol consumption, either.

According to a new survey of Americans by Detox.net:

- 36% of men and nearly 26% of women wouldn't give up alcohol for life even if it meant saving the life of a stranger,

- Almost 35% of daily drinkers wouldn't remain with their significant other if that person didn't approve of their alcohol use,

- 47.5% would rather give up coffee for a month than alcohol,

- 37.6% would rather give up sugar for a month than alcohol,

- 17.1% would rather give up sex for a month than alcohol, and

- The average person wouldn't give up alcohol for life for less than $365,458.

Fortunately, you don't have to give up alcohol or sugar completely. Just subtract some of each, and add some fiber, to see and feel the results you want.

Alcohol and Fructose - Pick Your Poison

Alcohol (also known as ethanol) and fructose make you fat in pretty much the same way, which is why sugar belly and beer belly are so closely related.

We make ethanol by fermenting sugar.

Once consumed, our brain metabolizes a small percentage of ethanol to give us a buzz (or make us drunk), but our liver does the real heavy lifting, and metabolizing ethanol takes precedence over everything else, including any stored fat which your body might otherwise have burned off.

Ethanol puts fat burning on the back burner, if you will.

The same is true of any fructose that you consume, except that *all* of it goes directly to your liver to be metabolized. The rest of your body wants nothing to do with it.

Why do ethanol and fructose make a beeline for the liver?

Because that's where the body metabolizes toxins or pseudo-toxins.

So, in that sense, you can pick your poison, alcohol or fructose.

They both tilt the Game of Hormones by assaulting your liver and setting off a chain reaction that makes you fat.

Alcohol is more dangerous (and arguably more fun) than fructose because some of it is metabolized in the brain right away. Whereas excess sugar consumption won't seriously harm or kill you immediately, you can do some major or even permanent damage to yourself by drinking way too much alcohol in one sitting. We've all heard the stories.

But remember this: In the long-term, excess consumption of sugar and alcohol cause many of the same serious health problems, including obesity in the form of sugar belly, beer belly, or some combination thereof.

That's why subtracting both of them from your diet makes so much sense.

Red Wine – Simply the Best

Drinking red wine in moderation leads to numerous health benefits.

Red wine provides 9.4% of your dietary reference intake of potassium, 5% for magnesium, and 4-9% for iron, but that's just for starters.

It also contains healthy antioxidants, including flavonoids and neoflavanoids, and one of the neoflavanoids—a chemical called **resveratrol** derived from the skin of grapes—may actually help to burn sugar-belly fat, reduce inflammation associated with obesity, fight cancer, and diminish your risk of heart disease.

(Tip: Pinot Noir contains the highest concentration of resveratrol among the red wines. So, unless you have a strong preference for another type, go for the Pinot.)

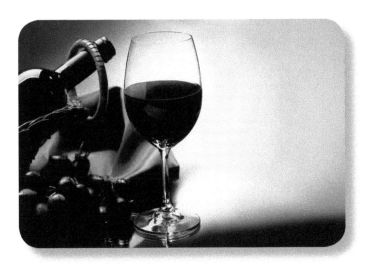

How cool is that?

White wine also has resveratrol, but red wine contains more because it ferments longer with the grape skins. Red wine also contains less fructose (0.5 to 1 gram per glass) than white wine (1.25 to 1.5 grams per glass), and we like that in step one of our process.

Tired of drinking red or white wine but want similar resveratrol benefits?

Order a glass of sparkling wine instead. Sparkling wines like Champagne from France, Prosecco from Italy or Cava from Spain contain resveratrol because they're made from red and white grapes. They also contain polyphenol antioxidants, which help to reduce the risk of heart disease and stroke by slowing the removal of nitric acid from the blood.

Many sparkling wines contain no more sugar than red wine, but some add sugar to balance out the bitterness or provide a more rounded flavor. Brut Zero and Brut Nature, for example, contain no added sugar and only about 0.5 to 1 gram per glass, and Prosecco contains only about 1 gram, but Demi-Sec sparkling wine contains approximately 8 grams (1 to 2 teaspoons of added sugar) per glass. Order wisely.

Sparkling wine also tends to cause hangovers and migraines more than regular wine, especially after the first glass or two. I don't know why that is, but it happens.

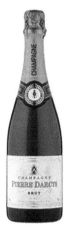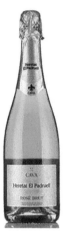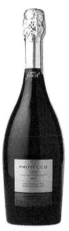

Finally, please don't confuse dessert wine with red, white, or sparkling wine. According to the USDA, dessert wine contains 8 grams of sugar per glass, but many brands include a lot more than that. A glass of Moscato contains 17 grams of sugar, for example.

Skip the dessert wine, please.

So, ideally, how much red, white, or sparkling wine should you drink?

Limit your consumption to one or two glasses a few nights a week if you want to lose weight. Less is more, especially for women and small men.

I know that a glass or two isn't much, and I don't want you to kick yourself if you blow it occasionally, but don't lose your focus, either.

Just do the best that you can, drink water in between alcoholic drinks (to combat dehydration and make you feel full), and remember that drinking in moderation will help you to flatten your sugar belly a whole lot faster.

Mixed Results

Whenever you consume an alcoholic beverage other than red wine, here's what happens:

- The ethanol in your drink punishes your liver, metabolism and sugar belly just like fructose, the worst of the sugars, does;

- Whereas 100% of the fructose that you consume travels directly to the liver because your body treats it like a toxin, about 80% of the ethanol that you consume in an alcoholic drink does the same thing. Your stomach and intestine break down another 10% of the ethanol, and the remaining 10% is metabolized by other organs, including your brain, which gives you the "buzz."

- Ethanol causes most of the same toxic effects as fructose in your Game of Hormones, including insulin resistance, leptin resistance, and metabolic syndrome; and

- Alcohol is metabolized directly into visceral, sugar-belly fat, just like fructose.

That's not a pretty picture, but if you consume alcoholic beverages besides red wine anyway—and I know that most of you will, at least from time to time—for goodness sakes, don't compound the problem by adding a sugary mixer to your drink.

Adding tonic, fruit juice or a sugary soda to your alcoholic beverage is one of the stupidest things you can do if you want to lose weight.

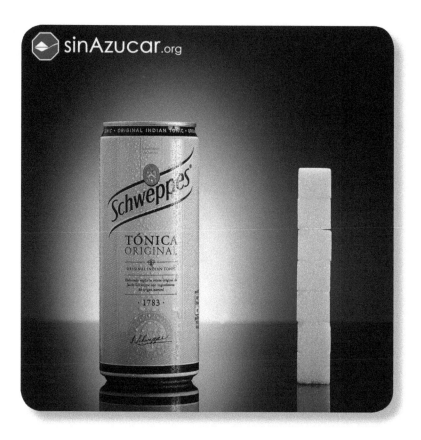

Drink your alcohol straight, or with soda water, instead.

What difference, at this point, does it make?

A big one.

Most booze consumed straight contains zero or near-zero grams of sugar. Your body still has to metabolize the ethanol, most of which will convert to fat, but the damage ends there.

However, soon as you mix your drink with tonic, fruit juice, or a sugary soda, you've added a ton of sugar to the beverage, including fructose that's going to hit your liver along with the ethanol like a double whammy… and *really* make you fat.

Therefore, if you're going to consume an alcoholic beverage other than (red) wine for the resveratrol and other nutritional benefits, choose something toward the top of the following list:

Alcoholic beverage (by the glass)	Grams of sugar (Approx.)
Distilled/hard/straight liquor (vodka, gin, whiskey, rum, tequila)	0

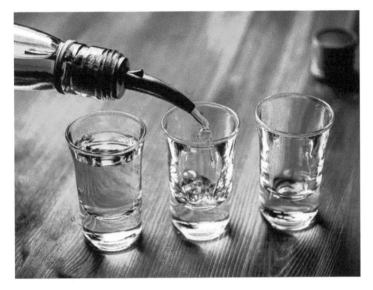

- Don't confuse distilled/hard liquor with sugary liqueurs, which often contain about 10 grams of sugar.

- Caution: Some rum producers add sugar to sweeten it. There's a brand in Medellin, Colombia called "Ron Medellin Anejo 8-year Extra Anejo," for example. It tastes great, but that's probably because of the added sugar, which is one reason why I don't drink it anymore.

Alcoholic beverage (by the glass)	Grams of sugar (Approx.)
Vodka soda	0

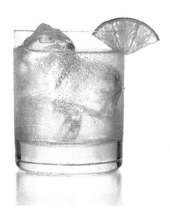

Beer	0 to 0.5

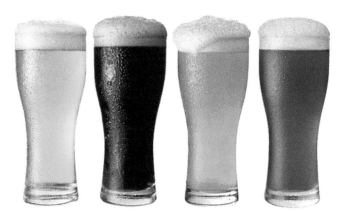

Alcoholic beverage (by the glass)	**Grams of sugar** (Approx.)

- Caution! Don't get excited and go pounding a bunch of beers because they're low in sugar. All else being equal, it's true that you're better off drinking a beer than many other alcoholic beverages with a more sugar (including cider beers), but watch out. Beer drinkers often fail to drink in moderation, which is bad for any type of alcohol consumption, and alcohol stimulates the appetite and insulin release, which screws up your Game of Hormones. Beer drinkers are also known to consume sugary, low-fiber "bar" food normally associated with it, like pizza, wings, other fried foods, or unhealthy snacks.

Red wine	0.5 to 1.0
Champagne (Brut Nature, Extra Brut, and Brut)	0.5 to 1.5
Prosecco	1.0
White wine	1.25 to 1.5
Aguardiente Liquor	2
Sweet Champagne (Extra Dry, Dry, Sec, and Demi-Sec)	2.8 to 8.3

- "Doux" sweet Champagne contains a lot more sugar than other types and should be avoided.

Daiquiri	3.4
Croft Original Sherry	9.5

Alcoholic beverage (by the glass)	**Grams of sugar** (Approx.)
Jägermeister (a shot)	12

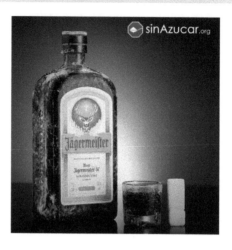

Gin and tonic	14 to 18

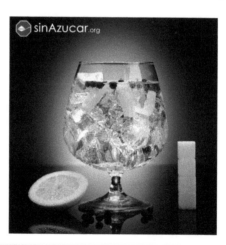

Bourbon Old Fashioned	15
Moscow Mule	15
Whiskey Sour	16 to 21

Alcoholic beverage (by the glass)	Grams of sugar (Approx.)
Martini	17
Margarita (depending on the contents and glass size)	17 to 31
Bailey's Irish Cream (3.38 ounces)	20

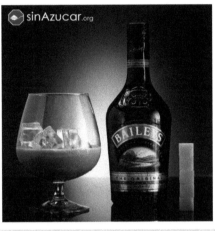

Bulmers Original Cider	20.5
Cosmopolitan	22

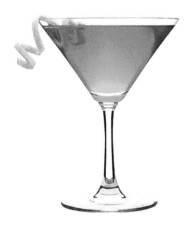

Alcoholic beverage (by the glass)	Grams of sugar (Approx.)
Angry Orchard Crisp Apple (Hard Cider)	24
Mojito (depending on glass size)	25 to 37
Rum and Coke	27.5 to 30
Pina Colada (depending on glass size)	27.5 to 43
Vodka Cranberry	30
Strawberry Daiquiri	33
Mike's Hard Lemonade	32
Jack and Coke	33

- I used to drink these all the time. Not anymore.

Long Island Iced Tea (depending on glass size)	39 to 60

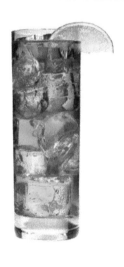

Alcoholic beverage (by the glass)	Grams of sugar (Approx.)
Four Loko	60

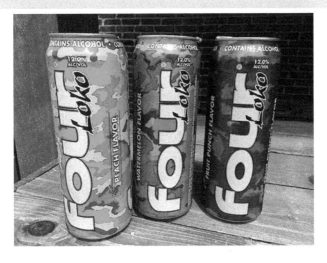

One more tip before we move on to the last chapter:

If you drink excessively on a particular day, consider a mini-fast to even the score. That's what I do. I eat nothing and drink only water and coffee for about 12 hours (including 8 hours of sleep).

When you deprive your body of food during a mini-fast or intermittent fast, it goes into a ketogenic state and starts burning some stored fat instead.

The Ketogenic diet is based on this principle. It's a great way to lose weight quickly, and some people swear by it, but it's not a long-term, sustainable solution to sugar belly for me and many others, and it's no fun. I don't want to count and cut my carbs so drastically or worry about calories or portion sizes, and I don't have to if I take three simple steps - subtract sugar, add fiber, and subtract alcohol.

That's the Sugar Belly Secret to healthy, sustainable weight loss, but you can double down by doing something else that I love to do, exercise.

Exercise is optional if you're consuming real, healthy, naturally slimming food and beverages by following the simple guidelines in this book.

But Chapter 6 will explain why adding at least some sort of exercise to your weight-loss program makes so much sense, and why I strongly recommend it.

CHAPTER 6

Double Down with Exercise

Very few people know my true P90X story—what *really* happened.

Frankly, I wouldn't have survived the first 30 days, let alone appear as a cast member in one of the P90X videos and an early success story in infomercials, if I hadn't changed my diet to something akin to the Sugar Belly Secret shortly after the program began.

On the first day of the P90X test group in Santa Monica, CA years ago, I knew my soft, 41-year old body (including a chronic bad back and varying degrees of sciatic nerve pain), wouldn't make it through 90 days of extreme exercise if I got hurt or sick at any point along the way, and I was determined not to let either of those two things happen.

But I was literally falling apart after the first 10 to 14 days of the program. When I brought this to the attention of Tony Horton (the fitness guru behind P90X who was teaching the classes) and a few others, they quickly realized that my diet at the time—I ate like a typical, stressed-out attorney—wasn't adequate and recommended that I either cook at home or order fresh, unprocessed food from a local food delivery service.

Since I wasn't about to start cooking, and I certainly wasn't going to embarrass myself by being one of the first to quit the test group, I started paying a company to deliver all my meals and snacks to my law office for the remainder of the program. (The producers of P90X, Beachbody, didn't have their own food delivery service.)

That was one of the smartest decisions I've ever made.

I felt and looked better almost immediately, and my final results were remarkable:

- My weight dropped from 181 pounds to 173 pounds;
- My body fat dropped from 14.3% to 8.7%; and
- My waistline shrunk from 33 inches to 30 inches.

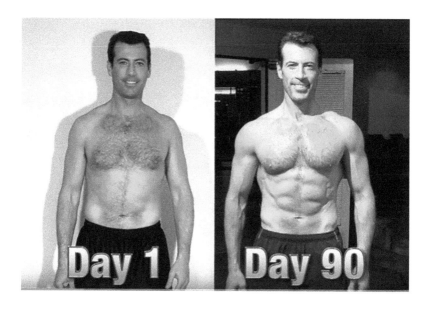

All good, right?

Well, not exactly. I may not look skinny in the Day 90 photo above because it was taken immediately after my last full-body workout when I was pumped up—unlike the Day 1 photo—but I was. I'm almost 6'2" tall, and I wanted to lose some belly fat during P90X, but I figured I'd replace it with heavier muscle, not shrink to 173 pounds.

I was fit, but I didn't add enough muscle to compensate for the fat loss.

To be fair, P90X isn't customized. It's a one-size-fits-all exercise program on DVDs (and now the Internet), where results will vary, but I learned the hard way that 173 pounds— 6-pack or no 6-pack—isn't a good look on a guy as tall as me.

How can I say that? Let me tell you a little story.

A couple of days after the P90X test group ended, I went to a bar in Santa Monica, CA with another guy who'd just completed the program and waited for a hot English girl to show up. I had a crush on her for years without much to show for it, but I thought my new P90X body would turn the tables. This was going to be my night.

I was leaning against the bar when she showed up, and I remember watching her walk toward me in what seemed to be slow motion. It was something out of a movie. She looked stunningly beautiful and excited to be there, but that all changed as she came closer.

She looked at me with a pained expression and said, "What happened? Are you alright? Have you been sick?" Taken aback, I said, "What are you talking about? I just completed a new, 90-day extreme home fitness program. I'm in the best shape of my life."

She wasn't impressed. "But you look so gaunt, like you're ill or something. I don't like it. You need to start eating more and drinking again. Excuse me... Bartender!"

That hurt. I had feelings for this girl and jumped through all of the P90X hoops for nothing, or at least that's how it felt. I looked *worse* in her eyes.

I wish I could say that I handled the let-down maturely, but I didn't. I made a rude, highly defensive remark and left.

Several days later, I called to apologize. She graciously forgave me, said she understood, and tried to make me feel better with an explanation that went something like this: "I'm sorry I hurt your feelings. I didn't mean to.

You always look handsome. It's just that, when I saw you, you reminded me of a close friend of mine who died recently of AIDS."

Ouch. AIDS?!

I took it better this time, but it still felt like a kick in the balls.

These days, I keep lean and healthy with the Sugar Belly Secret, and I exercise 5 or 6 times a week, but I don't overdo it.

I don't need extreme exercise programs, and neither do you.

If you like P90X, Insanity, CrossFit, or whatever, by all means go for it. I'm not trying to discourage you in any way, but you can lose your sugar belly for good without them.

In fact, if you exercise to burn calories rather than concentrating on the quality of those calories, you're setting yourself up for disappointment.

Think about it. To burn off the calories in a McDonald's Big Mac, large fries and large Coke, an average-sized man would have to run for 2 hours and 21 minutes or walk for 4 hours and 38 minutes. Similarly, to burn off the calories in a Starbucks Venti Java Chip Frappuccino blended coffee with 2% milk, an average-sized woman would have to do yoga for more than 2 hours or bike for 46 minutes.

Does that sound like a solid weight-loss plan to you? Hardly.

Forget about the calorie counting. Control the quality of your calories instead with the Sugar Belly Secret. Then, if you'd like to flatten your belly faster and significantly improve your overall health and fitness, add exercise to your daily routine. It burns fat, improves insulin sensitivity, builds healthy muscle, and perhaps most importantly, reduces your stress (cortisol) at at time when most of us would love to be a little more peaceful, carefree, and happy.

Feel the Burn

Exercise won't shrink your sugar belly if you don't subtract sugar, add fiber, and subtract alcohol from your diet, but it can greatly expedite a sugar-belly breakthrough if you play it smart.

Here's a surefire sugar-belly hack, for example, that I hope you'll try:

Do some type of cardiovascular exercise for at least 30 minutes first thing in the morning *on an empty stomach*. You can have coffee or water beforehand, but no smoothies or food.

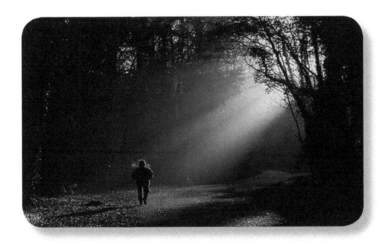

It works like a charm, and here's why:

When you wake up in the morning, you've effectively been fasting for 8 hours or however long you were resting. Consequently, your body doesn't have a ready source of carbs to use as energy when you start exercising before you eat. So it burns your stored fat for energy instead.

The low-carb Ketogenic diet is based on this fat-burning principle, and there's no better time to apply it than first thing in the morning.

Not a morning person? No worries. There's a Plan B.

Working out later in the day burns fat too, albeit not as rapidly and efficiently as doing it before breakfast.

Moreover, exercise of any kind builds muscle, which burns fat stored around the muscles themselves, as well as your liver and belly. It also improves insulin sensitivity, which leads to reduced insulin levels, and that's exactly what you want because excess insulin makes you fat.

Exercise actually burns two types of fat, visceral (intra-organ or sugar belly) fat and subcutaneous (big butt) fat.

Visceral fat jeopardizes your health and fitness more because it ends up where it doesn't belong – most notably, your waistline – and leads to inflammation, insulin resistance, obesity, metabolic syndrome, and the long list of potentially deadly diseases and conditions associated with it.

But there's a silver lining: Visceral fat is the first to go when you lose weight—that's right, your sugar belly will shrink before your big butt does—and it responds well to regular exercise that elevates your heart rate.

Subcutaneous fat, on the other hand, is healthier and much harder to lose, but regular exercise can burn off some of that too. All the more reason to do it.

Pump Up

Why wasn't I able to build enough muscle during the P90X test group to compensate for the fat loss and keep my weight at a reasonable level?

Diets typically result in the loss of more muscle than fat unless the dieter does enough exercise to maintain and build muscle along the way.

In my case, I was doing the Shoulders & Arms workout and other exercise routines to build muscle, but I was losing muscle too by dieting and doing a lot more strenuous cardio than usual. (If you've ever tried P90X Plyometrics, you know what I mean.)

In hindsight, I would have fared better by doing more weightlifting and less cardio, and eating even more healthy food to help prevent muscle loss, but I was learning on the fly, and so was everyone else. That's what happens in a test group.

Some things work; others don't. You do the best that you can, hope for the best, and learn from your mistakes.

I'm grateful for my P90X transformation and hope it doesn't sound otherwise, but I no longer allow dieting or cardiovascular activity to turn me into sickly stick figure with abs.

Instead, I double down on the Sugar Belly Secret with exercise to build muscle while burning fat at a healthy, sustainable rate, and I hope you do the same... even if you don't have to.

But there's another reason to exercise, and it's arguably the most important one: it reduces stress (cortisol) better than anything else, or at least I think so.

Peace Be with You

My descent from P90X Joe to Average Joe began long before my first bout with vertigo and really accelerated while working in a highly stressful environment as a patent litigation analyst in South Florida.

It started out as a cool job, and the company grew by leaps and bounds during my tenure, but then it got weird for everyone except the boss, who didn't change for the better in response to success. I tried not to take it personally, but at some point, just showing up for work was stressful.

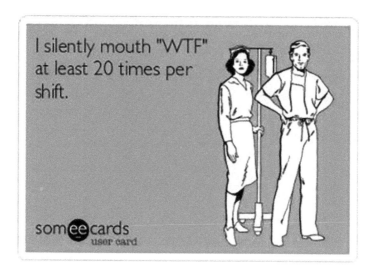

I didn't fall apart overnight, but I slowly let myself go. I ate poorly and stopped working out regularly. I worked long, unpredictable hours and didn't sleep well. And it showed from head to toe. I was pale, sickly, fat, and very unhappy about it.

At some point, I almost resigned myself to it.

But then I resigned from the job, instead.

It wasn't easy giving up the salary and benefits to become an aspiring author and producer, but saying goodbye to the stress of that job was another one of the best decisions I've ever made. Life is too short to accept a thoroughly unpleasant work environment if there's a reasonable alternative, and there usually is, even if it takes a leap of faith to get there.

I'm sure you've dealt with equally if not more stressful situations in your own life and know the feeling, whether the pressure arose from business, financial, or personal issues. (Coping with the loss of a loved one, especially a child, is obviously far worse, for example.)

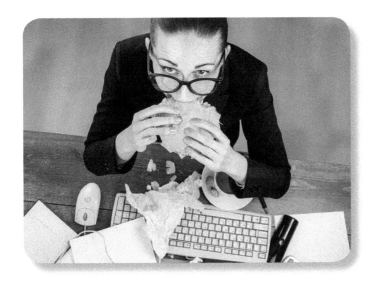

Of course, we can't eliminate all stress from our lives, and sometimes it's just the kick in the rear we need to do something brave, loving, or otherwise great. But stress is a killer if we don't respond to it properly and effectively.

As you know from our discussion in Chapter 2, cortisol is your stress hormone in the Game of Hormones, and excess cortisol leads to insulin resistance (that is, too much fat-producing insulin), consumption of comfort foods, and sugar-belly fat, all of which greatly increase the likelihood of obesity, metabolic syndrome and/or premature death.

And you can fight back by reducing your stress through meditation, yoga, more sleep, or maybe even quitting a lousy job like I did.

That's all good, but exercise reduces stress and the resulting release of cortisol into your system *more simply, inexpensively, and effectively than anything else,* and you enjoy the other benefits—burning fat, building healthy muscle, looking better—as a bonus.

A new study also suggests that exercise may increase your self-control when it comes to avoiding sugary food and beverages. Scientists are still trying to figure out exactly why this occurs, but I suspect that subjects who exercised simply weren't as likely to stress out and reach for comfort food.

Pretty cool, right? You bet.

Reducing stress through exercise will help you execute the Sugar Belly Secret more easily, naturally, and consistently, while making you healthier, stronger, and more far attractive in the process.

Conclusion

It's time to stop *reacting* to your sugar belly with trendy diets, exercise programs, exercise equipment, and weight-loss surgeries that produce short-term gains and long-term disappointment. Yo-yo results like that lead to cynicism and self-doubt and, in some cases, the skinny tease is almost worse than never trying at all.

As this book has demonstrated, there's a new, natural, simple, *proactive* strategy for losing weight and permanently transforming your life.

You don't need to obsess over counting calories, carbs or healthy fats, portion sizes, or even exercise.

And you aren't stuck with an unhealthy sugar belly or worsening metabolic syndrome for life just because you're currently overweight, obese, old, sickly, or just losing your edge, like I did after my P90X glory days.

You can start losing your sugar belly right now.

All you need to do is tweak your diet with 3 simple steps:

1. Subtract sugar,
2. Add fiber, and
3. Subtract alcohol.

That's the Sugar Belly Secret.

You don't have to completely eliminate sugar and alcohol from your diet, either. Less is more, but this weight-loss system doesn't require perfection or extreme measures.

You certainly don't have to eat fiber all day, either. A little goes a long way, and too much fiber will land you in the restroom for a reality check, anyway. (Your body will tell you when you've overdone it on the fiber, amigos, and I speak from experience on that one.)

And, while I haven't spent much time talking about "fats," it goes without saying that you should avoid fake, processed "trans fats." I didn't spend a chapter on it because it's become common knowledge, and food companies have already begun removing it from most of what they produce.

Stick with real food, including healthy fats like avocado, nuts, cheese, bacon, and coconut oil, apply the Sugar Belly Secret, and you'll be fine.

Once you realize that the food and beverage industries have adulterated our food supply by adding tons of sugar and removing fiber from almost everything, often surreptitiously, you can do the opposite and begin turning the tables almost immediately.

If you think some government agency is going to intervene by compelling companies to offer healthier food, think again. There's too much money to be made or saved by hiding the inconvenient truth from you, and it's much easier to blame you for not being smart or disciplined enough to resolve the problem than make it easier for you to do so.

It's up to you to outsmart the system, but you can do it with the Sugar Belly Secret and reap the benefits for a lifetime.

Reducing your consumption of sugar will reduce insulin resistance, adding fiber will diminish those fat-making insulin rushes, and drinking less alcohol or making smarter choices in that regard (red wine in particular) will help your body spend more time burning fat and less time storing it.

You will see and feel the difference as soon as you begin "un-processing" your diet by adding fiber while subtracting sugar and alcohol. After just a few simple modifications to your existing diet, you'll be consuming real food and beverages with higher-quality calories that naturally lead to weight loss.

And here's the kicker:

The Sugar Belly Secret is remarkably simple, manageable, and sustainable.

That's why, in my humble opinion, it's your best long-term solution.

As the saying goes, the best plan is one you can stick to, and you can definitely stick to this one. All you need to do is add and subtract.

If you want to expedite and maximize your results while building some healthy, fat-burning muscle and reducing stress, you can double down by adding one more thing, exercise.

Exercise is optional, but it complements the Sugar Belly Secret perfectly.

The choice is yours.

You can let the Sugar Belly Secret work its magic in a natural, sustainable way by making a few minor changes in the way you eat and live.

Or, you can ignore it and continue doing things that don't work for you in the long term and never will.

If you're not ready to try my new weight-loss system today, I respect your decision, but I hope I've planted a seed that will grow into something special someday.

Success leaves clues, and the Sugar Belly Secret is based on those clues.

I make mistakes all the time, but I watch what successful people do, learn from them, and follow in their footsteps when it makes sense to do so. I love to do my own thing, but there's no point in reinventing the wheel. I'd rather stand on the shoulders of giants and invite others to join me up there. That's why I wrote this book.

In a nutshell, the Sugar Belly Secret is about taking the best of the best low-carb and high-carb diets and distilling it all down to what really matters. Many of these diets work. I'm not claiming otherwise, and I'm especially fond of Keto and other low-carb diets. But they're too hard, extreme, complicated, and potentially hazardous to serve as a long-term solution.

The Sugar Belly Secret is different. It's more concerned about lasting, long-term improvement in your health, fitness, and appearance than short-term interventions that give you a taste of success before cruelly snatching it away, and I did my best to explain it as clearly as I could.

I hope you found this book entertaining as well because there's no reason why we shouldn't have a little fun together along the way. This is a weight-loss program, not a bombing mission over 'Nam.

Plus, stressing out over your sugar belly is only going to make it worse.

My departed grandmother, Katherine ("Kitty") Howe, was one of the most lovable and truly delightful people I've ever known.

Everyone saw and felt how special she was, and it didn't take long.

One day in her home, I asked, "Gram, what's the secret to life?"

She just giggled, thought about it for a second or two, and said, "Oh … just be happy and laugh a lot!"

I remember being slightly disappointed. That's it? Then it hit me.

By thinking and living like that, she developed a *habit* of laughter and happiness.

I never forgot it and try not to lose my sense of humor or joy, especially when it comes to basic things like eating, drinking, and exercising.

Maybe that's why the Sugar Belly Secret works so well for me.

It's more than just simple, logical, natural, and sustainable.

You can lose weight, build muscle, and significantly improve your overall health and fitness… with a laugh and a smile.

So, are you ready to lose your sugar belly?

Well, as they say here in Medellin, "Hagale pues!" (Do it, then!)

I'll be there to guide you every step of the way to a successful outcome.

ALSO BY JOE BOVINO

For even faster and more remarkable results, order Joe Bovino's complete Sugar Belly Secret weight-loss system.

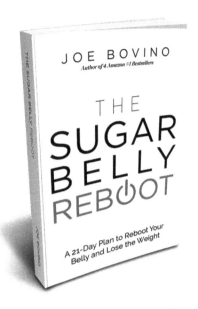

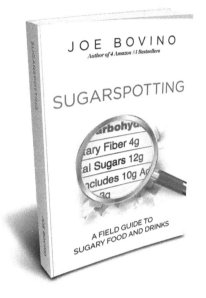

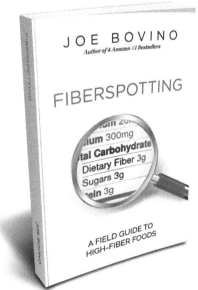

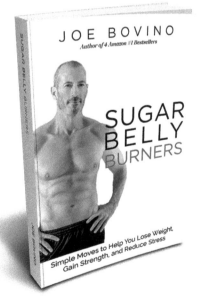

Available only at

www.TheSugarBellySecret.com

Notes

Introduction

Smyth, Chris, "Poor diet 'biggest health risk' as obesity deaths rise," *The Australian,* September 16, 2017. http://www.theaustralian.com.au/news/world/the-times/poor-diet-biggest-health-risk-as-obesity-deaths-rise/news-story/6fdf155d8ccecd07dfd017faf78cd3e1.

Glenza, Jessica. "Cancers Linked to Excess Weight Make up 40% of All US Diagnoses, Study Finds." *The Guardian*, Guardian News and Media, 3 Oct. 2017, www.theguardian.com/society/2017/oct/03/cancer-obesity-weight-us-study.

Lustig, Robert H., *Fat Chance: Beating the Odds Against Sugar, Processed Foods, Obesity and Disease*, Plume 2014

Lustig, Robert H. "Sugar: The Bitter Truth." University of California Television, 30 July 2009, www.youtube.com/watch?v=dBnniua6-oM.

Jacoby, Richard and Baldalomar, Raquel, *Sugar Crush: How to Reduce Inflammation, Reverse Nerve Damage, and Reclaim Good Health*, Harper Wave, 2016

Taubes, Gary, *The Case Against Sugar*, Knopf, 2016.

Zinczenko, David, *Zero Sugar Diet: The 14-Day Plan to Flatten Your Belly, Crush Cravings, and Help You Keep Lean for Life*, Ballantine Books, 2016.

Chapter 1: The Scoop on Added Sugar

Lustig, Robert H., *Fat Chance: Beating the Odds Against Sugar, Processed Foods, Obesity and Disease*, Plume 2014

Lustig, Robert H. "Sugar: The Bitter Truth." University of California Television, 30 July 2009, www.youtube.com/watch?v=dBnniua6-oM.

Jacoby, Richard and Baldalomar, Raquel, *Sugar Crush: How to Reduce Inflammation, Reverse Nerve Damage, and Reclaim Good Health*, Harper Wave, 2016

Taubes, Gary, *The Case Against Sugar*, Knopf, 2016.

Zinczenko, David, *Zero Sugar Diet: The 14-Day Plan to Flatten Your Belly, Crush Cravings, and Help You Keep Lean for Life*, Ballantine Books, 2016.

"Adult Obesity in the United States." *The State of Obesity*. Trust for America's Health and the Robert Wood Johnson Foundation, August 31, 2017. https://stateofobesity.org/adult-obesity/

Boseley, Sarah. "Sugar, Not Fat, Exposed as Deadly Villain in Obesity Epidemic." *The Guardian*, 20 Mar. 2013. https://www.theguardian.com/society/2013/mar/20/sugar-deadly-obesity-epidemic

The GBD 2015 Obesity Collaborators, "Health Effects of Overweight and Obesity in 195 Countries over 25 Years." *New England Journal of Medicine*, 6 July 2017. http://www.nejm.org/doi/full/10.1056/NEJMoa1614362#t=article

Bedard, Paul. "Obesity Becomes Worldwide Epidemic, US Is the Fattest." *Washington Examiner*, 26 July 2017. http://www.washingtonexaminer.com/obesity-becomes-worldwide-epidemic-us-is-the-fattest/article/2629712

"I'm Not Fat... I'm Evolved • r/CringeAnarchy." *Reddit*, citing an article from The Sun. Retrieved on September 9, 2017 at www.reddit.com/r/CringeAnarchy/comments/6yanls/im_not_fat_im_evolved.

Chapter 2: Game of Hormones

Steen, Juliette. "So, This Is Exactly How Sugar Makes Us Fat." *HuffPost*, 21 Apr. 2017. http://www.huffingtonpost.com.au/amp/2017/04/20/so-this-is-exactly-how-sugar-makes-us-fat_a_22046969/

Johnston, Ian, "'Catastrophic' lack of sleep in modern society is killing us, warns leading sleep scientist," *The Independent*, 24 September 2017, www.independent.co.uk/news/sleep-deprivation-epidemic-health-effects-tired-heart-disease-stroke-dementia-cancer-a7964156.html?amp.

Chapter 3: Subtract Added Sugar

Lustig, Robert H., *Fat Chance: Beating the Odds Against Sugar, Processed Foods, Obesity and Disease*, Plume 2014

Zinczenko, David, *Zero Sugar Diet: The 14-Day Plan to Flatten Your Belly, Crush Cravings, and Help You Keep Lean for Life*, Ballantine Books, 2016.

"Sugar Delirium Blog - Beverages." *How Much Sugar in Sodas and Beverages?*, *Sugar Stacks*, Retrieved on 2 Sept. 2017 at http://www.sugarstacks.com/beverages.htm.

'Carbonated Soft Drinks – Pepsi," *Official Site for PepsiCo Beverage Information | Product.* Retrieved on October 24, 2017 at www.pepsicobeveragefacts.com/Home/Product?formula=35005%2A26%2A01-01&form=RTD&size=20.

Jehring, Andy. "LESS IS MORE. Low Calorie Diet Drinks and Foods 'Trick the Brain into Making You Fatter' - and Could Trigger Diabetes." *The Sun*, 11 Aug. 2017. https://www.thesun.co.uk/living/4219398/low-calorie-diet-drinks-foods-fatter-diabetes

Ferro, Shaunacy, "How Much Sugar Is in Your Pizza? Way More Than You'd Think." *Mental Floss*, 18 Jan. 2017. http://mentalfloss.com/article/91033/how-much-sugar-your-pizza-way-more-youd-think

"Sugarstacks." *H2Operation*. Retrieved on September 15, 2017 at www.h2operation.org/sugarstacks.

Cardoza, Riley, "30 Sugariest Foods In America." *Eat This Not That*, 23 Aug. 2017. https://tinyurl.com/ya4wfcdp.

"Revelando El Azúcar Libre De Los Alimentos." *SinAzucar.org*. Retrieved on September 2, 2017 at www.sinazucar.org.

"Caffè Mocha." *Starbucks Coffee Company*. Retrieved on September 2, 2017 at https://www.starbucks.com/menu/drinks/espresso/caffe-mocha#size=121967&milk=63&whip=NA

"Dunkin' Donuts Nutrition Facts & Calorie Information: A Nutrition Guide to the Dunkin' Donuts Menu for Healthy Eating." *Nutrition-Charts.com*, 16 Feb. 2016, http://www.nutrition-charts.com/dunkin-donuts-nutrition-information./

"Labeling & Nutrition - Changes to the Nutrition Facts Label." *U S Food and Drug Administration Home Page*, Center for Food Safety and Applied Nutrition, June 19, 2017. https://www.fda.gov/Food/GuidanceRegulation/ GuidanceDocumentsRegulatoryInformation/LabelingNutrition/ ucm385663.htm

Benshosan, Olivia Tarantino & April. "The FDA Delays Deadline For New Nutrition Labels," *Eat This Not That*, 9 Oct. 2017, www.eatthis.com/fda-delays-new-nutriton-label/.

"How To Spot Sugar On Food Labels." *Hungry For Change*. Retrieved on September 2, 2017 at http://www.hungryforchange.tv/article/how-to-spot-sugar-on-food-labels

Mottl, Pooja R. "Food Labels: How to Spot Hidden Sugars." *The Huffington Post*, TheHuffingtonPost.com, 18 Jan. 2011, http://www.huffingtonpost. com/pooja-r-mottl/food-labels-hidden-sugars_b_808881.html

Wagstaff, Camilla, "What's REALLY in Your Food? A Guide to Reading Food Labels (+between the lines)." *I Quit Sugar*, 22 June 2016, https://iquitsugar.com/whats-really-food-guide-reading-food-labels-lines/

Chapter 4: Add Fiber

English, Nick, "The 16 Most Surprising High-Fiber Foods." *Greatist*, 23 September. 2013, https://greatist.com/health/surprising-high-fiber-foods

Anna. "10 Harmoniously High Fiber Foods." *ActiveBeat*, Retrieved on September 2, 2017 at http://www.activebeat.com/diet-nutrition/10-harmoniously-high-fiber-foods/

Steen, Juliette. "So, This Is Exactly How Sugar Makes Us Fat." *HuffPost*, 21 Apr. 2017, http://www.huffingtonpost.com.au/amp/2017/04/20/so-this-is-exactly-how-sugar-makes-us-fat_a_22046969/

Coles, Terri. "14 High-Fibre Foods You Should Be Eating Every Day." *HuffPost* Canada, 9 Dec. 2016, http://www.huffingtonpost.ca/2013/10/31/high-fibre-foods_n_4178239.html

House, Paul. "27 Beans and Legumes High in Fiber." *HealthAliciousNess*, 22 June 2017, https://www.healthaliciousness.com/articles/beans-legumes-high-in-fiber.php

Mayo Clinic Staff, "How Much Fiber Is Found in Common Foods?" *Mayo Clinic*, Mayo Foundation for Medical Education and Research, 8 Oct. 2015, http://www.mayoclinic.org/healthy-lifestyle/nutrition-and-healthy-eating/in-depth/high-fiber-foods/art-20050948

Mayo Clinic Staff, "The Do's and Don'ts of a Low-Fiber Diet." *Mayo Clinic*, Mayo Foundation for Medical Education and Research, 25 July 2017, www.mayoclinic.org/healthy-lifestyle/nutrition-and-healthy-eating/in-depth/low-fiber-diet/art-20048511.

"Sugary Cereals: Which Are the 10 'Worst?" *CBS News*, CBS Interactive, 7 Dec. 2011, www.cbsnews.com/pictures/sugary-cereals-which-are-the-10-worst/2.

"Cap'N Crunch." *FatSecret*, Retrieved on September 2, 2017 at www.fatsecret.com/calories-nutrition/generic/capn-crunch?portionid=15883&portionamount=1.000.

"Lucky charms: Cereals ready to eat, general mill," *Eat This Much*. Retrieved on October 11, 2017 at www.eatthismuch.com/food/view/lucky-charms,1031.

"Kellogg's Honey Smacks." *FatSecret*, Retrieved on September 2, 2017 at www.fatsecret.com/calories-nutrition/kelloggs/honey-smacks.

Gunnars, Kris. "11 Proven Health Benefits of Chia Seeds." *Healthline*, Healthline Media, 30 May 2017, www.healthline.com/nutrition/11-proven-health-benefits-of-chia-seeds.

Chapter 5: Subtract Alcohol

Henriques, Martha. "Alcoholism Epidemic in the USA: More than 1 in 8 Americans Are Now Alcoholics." *International Business Times UK*, 11 Aug. 2017, www.ibtimes.co.uk/alcoholism-epidemic-more-1-8-americans-are-now-alcoholics-1634315.

"What Would You Give Up for Alcohol?" *Detox.net*, 19 June 2017, www.detox.net/uncover/what-would-you-give-up-for-alcohol.

Rose, Brent. "The Nine Healthiest Alcoholic Drinks." *Gizmodo*, Gizmodo.com, 13 July 2012, http://gizmodo.com/5925820/the-nine-healthiest-alcoholic-drinks.

Wilson, Sara, "Can I Drink Alcohol When I Quit Sugar?" *I Quit Sugar.* Retrieved on September 2, 2017 at https://iquitsugar.com/faqs/can-i-drink-wine.

Schaefer, Anna. "Red Wine and Type 2 Diabetes: Is There a Link?" *Healthline*, 23 Nov. 2015, www.healthline.com/health/diabetes/red-wine-and-type-2-diabetes.

Munro, Angela. "Red Wine Ingredient Resveratrol May Boost Metabolism in Men." *Red Wine Ingredient Resveratrol May Boost Metabolism in Men | Health | The Earth Times*, www.earthtimes.org/health/red-wine-ingredient-resveratrol-boost-metabolism-men/1583/.

Millehan, Jan. "Connection Between Wine & Belly Fat." *Livestrong.com*, Leaf Group, 18 July 2017, www.livestrong.com/article/445668-connection-between-wine-belly-fat.

"HAMS: Harm Reduction for Alcohol: Carbs, Sugar, and Alcohol Content of Various Drinks." *HAMS: Harm Reduction for Alcohol.* Retrieved on September 2, 2017 at http://hams.cc/carbs/ .

"Champagne Sweetness Scale: From Brut to Doux." *Wine Folly*, 9 Apr. 2015. http://winefolly.com/review/how-much-sugar-in-brut-champagne/

Jones, Tegan, "Cheers To That! 8 Unexpected Benefits Of Champagne." *Lifehack*, 28 Mar. 2014, www.lifehack.org/articles/lifestyle/cheers-that-8-unexpected-benefits-champagne.html.

"How Much Sugar Is in Your Glass of Bubbly?" *Glass Of Bubbly*, 14 July 2017, www.glassofbubbly.com/much-sugar-glass-bubbly.

"Calories in Aguardiente Liquor," *Calories in Aguardiente Liquor - Calories and Nutrition Facts | MyFitnessPal.com.* Retrieved on October 11, 2017 at www.myfitnesspal.com/food/calories/aguardiente-liquor-358329756?v2=false.

"The Amazing Similarities Between This Toxic Sugar and Alcohol." *Mercola.com*, September 9, 2012. http://articles.mercola.com/sites/articles/archive/2012/09/09/ethanol-alcohol-and-fructose.aspx

"How Much Sugar Is In Your Alcoholic Drinks?" *BuzzFeedBlue*, 3 July 2015, www.youtube.com/watch?v=vGSKYt-G4Nw&sns=em.

"What's the 411 on Four Loko?" *Go Ask Alice!*, Columbia University in the City of New York. Retrieved on September 2, 2017 at http://goaskalice.columbia.edu/answered-questions/whats-411-four-loko

Victor, Anucyia, "How Much Sugar Does Your Drink REALLY Contain? From a Small White Wine to a Glass of Prosecco - We Reveal the Best and Worst Alcoholic Tipples." *Daily Mail Online*, Associated Newspapers, 22 June 2015, www.dailymail.co.uk/femail/food/article-3131012/We-reveal-sugar-alcoholic-drink-REALLY-contains.html.

Malnick, Edward. "Hidden Levels of Sugar in Alcohol Revealed." *The Telegraph*, Telegraph Media Group, 29 Mar. 2014, www.telegraph.co.uk/foodanddrink/10731418/Hidden-levels-of-sugar-in-alcohol-revealed.html.

Dangerfield, Maya. "The Hard Choice: Is Beer or Cider Better?" *Greatist*, 6 June 2016, https://greatist.com/health/beer-or-cider-healthier.

"Pina Colada." *FatSecret*. Retrieved on September 2, 2017 at www.fatsecret.com/calories-nutrition/generic/pina-colada.

Andersen, Charlotte Hilton. "How Many Calories Are In Your Favorite Cocktails?" *Shape Magazine*, 10 Dec. 2015, www.shape.com/healthy-eating/healthy-drinks/calorie-count-all-your-favorite-cocktails.

Duvauchelle, Joshua. "Does Drinking Beer Make You Fat?" *Livestrong.com*, Leaf Group, 18 Dec. 2013, www.livestrong.com/article/464684-does-drinking-beer-make-you-fat.

Zelman, Kathleen M. "The Truth About Beer and Your Belly." *WebMD*. Retrieved on September 2, 2017 at www.webmd.com/diet/features/the-truth-about-beer-and-your-belly#2.

Chapter 6: Double Down with Exercise

"P90X® Success Stories - P90X Extreme Home Fitness Workout Program." *Beachbody*, Retrieved on October 24, 2017 at www.beachbody.com/ product/p90x-success-stories-joeb.do.

Romano, Andrea. "Calculator Showing How Much Exercise It Takes to Burn off Fast Food Will Ruin Your Lunch Plans." *Mashable*, 4 Mar. 2016, http://mashable.com/2016/03/04/fast-food-work-out-calculator/#xg62KXWB5Pqs

Reynolds, Gretchen. "How Exercise Might Increase Your Self-Control." *The New York Times*, 27 Sept. 2017, www.nytimes.com/2017/09/27/well/move/ how-exercise-might-increase-your-self-control.html?mwrsm=Email.

"The Fallacies Of Fat." *NPR*, 11 Jan. 2013, www.npr.org/2013/01/11 /169144853/the-fallacies-of-fat.

CPSIA information can be obtained
at www.ICGtesting.com
Printed in the USA
BVHW011041090723
666908BV00018B/911